ROCK THE PINK

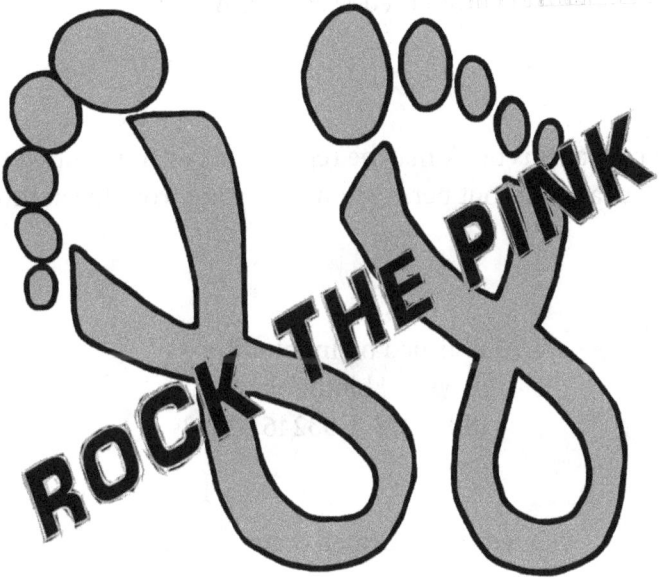

INKBLOT BOOKS

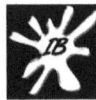

Rock The Pink

Published by Inkblot Books
www.inkblotbooks.com
ISBN 978-1-932461-31-2

Printed in the United States of America

ROCK THE PINK

K.A. THOMPSON

About This Book

Rock the Pink is part memoir, part what-it's-like guide. It grew from my 3 Day training blog, A Wabbit Walking, where I began journaling the minutiae of training for my first Susan G. Komen 3 Day for the Cure walk.

Some of you might want to skip right to information about the walk itself (Rock the Walk); because I have only participated in 3 DAy events thus far (but am taking on the Avon Walk in 2012 and possibly the MS Challenge Walk) what I describe is a 3 Day event, but after numerous discussions with other breast cancer walk participants, it became clear that much of what you'll find here covers the bases for other walk events.

In the first part of the book (which is pretty much about me) there are tips and hints within the narrative, so if you skipped to the second half, skimming over my musings might pay off a little.

At the back of the book are tips gathered from experienced 3 Day and Avon walkers.

Rock the Walk, my friends!

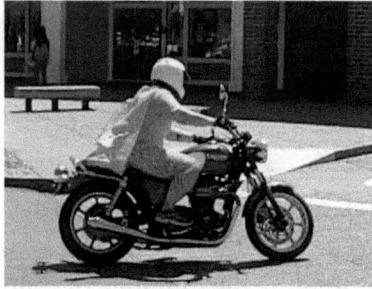

Trust me, you'll do just about anything to get donations...

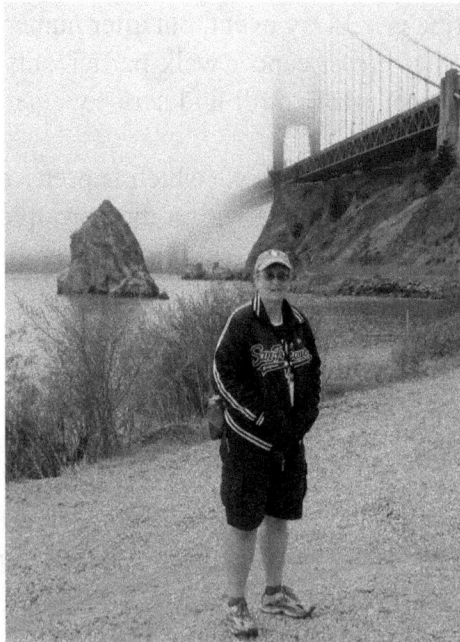

You get to see cool, stuff like the Golden Gate Bridge from both sides, as well as this view from the bottom.

Table of Contents

PREFACE

I didn't set out to write this book. Granted, I had notions of writing *a* book as I went about training for this walk, but I wasn't planning on writing anything other than blog entries to chronicle the whole experience. While I chewed through the training miles, planting one foot in front of the other, I had thoughts about my next novel percolating in my head; I mentally outlined the plot and visualized the setting, all while sweating from one mile to the next. I heard the dialog in my head. I also harbored a fear of talking to myself while I did this, and garnering a reputation around town of being that crazy lady who stumbles around talking to herself.

The blog, *A Wabbit Walking*, became my dumping ground for training minutiae; how far I walked, the condition of my feet and my battle with blisters, and I chronicled a few of the things I saw while walking around the tiny town of Dixon, California. I feared it was incredibly boring, but I was asking people to donate money to my fundraising effort, and for that they deserved some accountability on my part. If I wasn't holding up my end of the bargain? Well, they couldn't get their money back, but they could verbally ream me up one wall and down another if they so chose, and I would deserve it.

As every training mile faded behind me, when I wasn't mentally writing that novel, I found myself pondering what this walk really meant to me and what it might mean to other people. I had an idea of why and for whom I was training for an event that would have me slogging through sixty miles over a mere three days; on the surface, I was doing it because I had been invited to join a team and I do have a deeply seeded need to be liked, but I wondered what motivated other participants.

Ostensibly, I began this journey on May 7, 2010, when I received a comment on my cat's blog (yes, my cat has a blog. Shuddup. You probably read it every now and then.) from another blogger who had already participated in the walk several times. She'd done the San Francisco 3 Day in 2009 and was cheered on by several other cat bloggers; I probably would have been there with then, but while she was walking I was in the hospital getting my gall bladder yanked out. For 2010 some of those bloggers were joining her, and she extended an invitation to me to join them.

My initial reaction—one I didn't fire back in reply—was *are you freaking nuts? You want me to walk how far?*

Granted, I had planned on going into San Francisco to shake some metaphorical pom-poms, and had even considered wearing an outrageous costume and making an ass of myself, but personal participation was never on my radar. I was fat, out of shape, and had a laundry list of medical issues. Why would it be?

Still…I didn't leap to say no. I replied that I had to think about it; that was a lot of money to commit to—$2300—and I wanted to consult with my husband first. But "no" was the answer that was poised on the tip of my brain's tongue. It wasn't possible. Even if I could raise that much money, there was no way I would ever be able to walk twenty miles a day, three days running.

I headed to bed, resolved that in the morning I would (very politely) decline the invitation; I had reasons that were logical, reasons that were not excuses, reasons that would illicit "oh, of course" from most people.

Fibromyalgia.
Chronic Myofascial Pain Syndrome.
Arthritis of the lower spine.
Arthritis in both hips.
Diabetes Insipidus.
Hypothyroid.
Half a dozen other things resulting from a pituitary tumor.

Committing to training for a *sixty* mile walk? It would be foolish.

My resolve to decline waxed and waned all night. I couldn't walk even a mile without an incredible amount of discomfort; how could I be expected to work up to sixty? I lived with three chronic pain issues; if I did this I would just exacerbate them and could wind up in some serious trouble. I had issues from a pituitary tumor that had been removed in 2002; if my medications weren't working well, I could wind up with electrolytes completely screwed up and my blood running thick.

There was no way I could do this…

…unless I could.

What if I just gave the training a try? I could start the fundraising. As long as I didn't check into the walk on the first day, I wouldn't personally be responsible for covering the difference between what I'd raised and the minimum goal amount. How would I ever know if I didn't give it a go?

People who donated would surely understand if I fell short.

Right?

I could at least give it a shot.

But…the pain. I owned a damned wheelchair because of the pain. We'd stopped doing things we enjoyed because of the pain. Just thinking about it was sheer stupidity. And the money…what if I didn't raise enough but still felt like I had to check into the walk? That was a sizable chunk of change to cough up. And I'm borderline freakish about going new places alone…if Mike couldn't get that weekend off, going by myself would be pure torture.

But.

But.

But.

I tossed and turned all night. I absolutely didn't want to take on the risks that training for this walk would impose on me. And yet, I absolutely wanted to do it.

Mike told me when he got home from work in the morning—I had sent him a text message about it—that there was enough notice, so he'd be able to get the weekend off.

If I didn't raise enough money, he was fine with covering the difference.

I got online and fired a message off.

"I'm registering now before I change my mind."

Fifteen minutes later, as I sat in the living room with my laptop perched on my knees, I recall only one other thought.

What the hell did I just do?

0 To 60 In Just 13 Years
=or=
Me, me, and more me

Winter in North Dakota sucks. When it doesn't suck, it blows. If it's not sucking or blowing, it's gotten too cold to give a damn about anything, and certainly too cold to be worrying about sucking or blowing.

The oddest thing about being in North Dakota during a sucking blowfest of a wicked winter?

We were there by choice.

Oh yeah, it was mostly my bright idea. We had been stationed at Scott Air Force Base in Illinois and it was time to consider the realities of facing another Permanent Change of Station (which happens roughly every three years, making one wonder what part of "permanent" doesn't the government understand?) Rather than risk the Powers That Be having the lone choice about where we would next land—because that carried the risk of being sent to Outer Bumfark in the Third Circle of Hell located just under the Arctic Polar cap—we decided to create a dream list to be submitted for official consideration.

They really do call it a dream list. I think that's mostly because some middle aged guy who's aching to finally retire sits there and looks at all the exotic places people want to be stationed—places like Colorado and California and Inner

Bumfark—and snorts derisively while chuckling, "You're dreaming."

For the life of me, I can't remember why, but I desperately wanted to go someplace with snow. I wanted real snow, not just flurries that would occasionally settle into a microscopic layer of an almost-dusting on the grass. I wanted snow we could play in, snow worthy of wicked snowball fights and deep, artistic snow angels.

North Dakota certainly seemed to fit that criterion.

So the Spouse Thingy (don't look at me like that…it's an affectionate term. I swear. He doesn't mind.) filled out his dream list with North Dakota placed at the top, and sooner rather than later the word came down.

"Congratulations, you're going to Grand Forks Air Force Base."

I believe there was quite a bit of snark in that, but I can't be sure.

~

There are four seasons in North Dakota.

Almost Winter
Winter
Hey Remember Winter, and
How the Heck Can There Be This Many Mosquitos?

We arrived in late July, the thick of mosquito season. It was warm and humid, something not unfamiliar—we'd been stationed in San Antonio twice and were uncomfortably familiar with 100 degree temperatures wetted down with 95% humidity—but I don't think any of us expected to exit the car and be slapped in the face with an invisible wet washcloth.

Welcome to Grand Forks.

Splat.

Oh, I could live with the thick, damp air. I could even learn to tolerate being eaten alive by the swarms of tiny mosquitos that seemed to aim straight for me, ignoring the Spouse Thingy and our thirteen-year-old son, Curt. I could live with it because snow was on the horizon. Granted, it might be four or five months, but dammit, I was going to get my snow. Lots of white, fluffy, Northern American snow; the idea of it made settling into an ancient duplex with tiny bedrooms on the Air Force base tolerable, and I pondered the wonder of it.

We could learn to ski.

Decorating for Christmas would be wonderful! With real snow, our Christmas decorations would be bright and shiny and loaded with holiday spirit and would give all the neighbors warm fuzzies.

We could even look for someplace to rent a snowmobile. There would be zooming through fields of snow, our cheeks and noses turning red and tiny ice crystals would form on our eyelashes.

We were going to have real snow, and I was thrilled.

You know what?

Be careful what you wish for.

~

Our first winter in Grand Forks was filled with the wonder of snow. In fact, it was filled with so much wonder that a record 117" of the damned stuff fell. One hundred seventeen inches. And in North Dakota that crap sticks to the ground. It's unlike other areas where five or six inches falls, the kids play in it for a couple of days, and it melts away.

No, in North Dakota the snow falls and stays there. A few days later, more of it drops from the sky, and the next thing you know the wind is whipping it around and you can't see two feet in front of you, and you're trying to get the dog to go out in the back yard, but he's not stupid. It's freaking cold and he wants what's left of his neutered junk to stay right where it is, not freeze off and drop into a drift where it will remain until the spring thaw.

It would be nice to have someone else to blame for us being there during the winter of 1996-1997, but it was my idea.

Well, I can also blame the Air Force, because there's nothing permanent about a change of station and we only requested it because there was no way they were going to let us stay in Illinois.

Fine.

It's Uncle Sam's fault.

We'll go with that.

~

January 31, 1997.

Two days post ice storm.

Payday was a day early. Curt needed new contacts and they were waiting for pickup in the optical shop at Walmart. I needed new jeans to cover my ever-expanding backside, but there was no way in hell I was buying a pair of the high-waisted just-under-the-boobs Mom Jeans sold at the base exchange. And there was Red Lobster; having to go into town for the contacts and jeans was a ready-made excuse to go out for lunch and spend money we really couldn't afford on trucked-in "fresh" fish and Cajun chicken linguini, and a few of those killer cheese biscuits.

Curt had needed the contacts for three days, but the advent of the ice storm closed the highway and kept us tucked away safely on the air force base. He was a resourceful kid and capable of figuring out what to do to make too-long-worn contacts last a few more days. It wasn't like he was going anywhere he would need good vision, anyway.

The storm passed, the roads were plowed, the sun came out, angels began to sing the Hallelujah Chorus, and two days after the highway had been shut down it was re-opened.

Now, we're not completely lacking in intelligence. We didn't just hop into the truck and speed towards the front gate of the base, heading into town at ninety miles an hour. We looked around; the streets on base had been plowed and were ice-free and dry. School had not been canceled, which meant the buses taking the older kids to the high school in town had to take the same highway we would need to drive on. Other people were out and about.

It seemed safe enough.

The roads off base were more wet than on, but they'd been plowed and looked just fine. Mike (the aforementioned Spouse Thingy; I won't drive you nuts by calling him that all the time) took it easy and drove well under the speed limit, staying in the right hand lane to allow the gutsier drivers to pass on the left. There was no hurry; Walmart, the mall, and Red Lobster weren't going anywhere.

Yes, the roads looked fine.

Wet, but fine.

Now, this should have been major foreshadowing. It's winter in North Dakota. Cold. Freezing cold. The road looks wet. It looks fine, but is clearly wet.

Go ahead, say it out loud.

Duh.

A mile and a half from the base we were passed by a pickup truck that wasn't speeding—I doubt the driver was doing more than 45-50—but the wake of air generated by the passing truck and the stretch of (wet-but-fine!) black ice we were unwittingly upon sent our small pickup truck fishtailing. It started with the tail-fin shake of a startled guppy and rapidly escalated to the throttle of a pissed off Great White Shark. Before Mike could get the truck under control it spun around 360 degrees, and we were headed for the side of the road.

Normally the sides of Highway 2 slope down into a ditch, but at the peak of winter they were filled with hard packed snow and were covered with a silky sheen of ice. The truck's tires hit the icy edge between pavement and snow, caught, and we started to roll.

"Shit, shit, shit," was the only thing Mike could sputter.

I saw the snow rushing at us as the truck began to roll and felt an odd slice of calm. "It's all right."

One way or the other, dead or alive, I was pretty sure in that moment that everything was all right. Whatever was going to happen was going to happen, and it would be all right.

It was my Moment of Bullshit Zen. And it made sense at the time. Yeah, we might die, but hey! It would be all-freaking-right.

Had it been summer, we'd have probably been bending over, prepping to become death's newest bitches. The tires would have hit the edge of the road and the truck would have rolled with a snap, the cab slamming into hard packed dirt before bouncing into the ditch, where it would be crushed in even further. That the ditch was filled with snow probably saved our lives. We didn't bounce; we rolled first onto the side of the truck, and then almost lazily it kept turning over until we were upside down. The truck was totaled, but the snow filled ditch was probably what saved our lives.

After a few moments of hanging upside down, the shattered windshield mere millimeters from our faces, we carefully unclasped our seatbelts and crawled out the passenger door—the driver's side door jammed too deeply into the snow to budge—and we were just glad to be alive, amazed that neither of us was hurt.

It was bitterly cold—January in Grand Forks, don'tcha know—and while we waited for the police, a dozen other drivers pulled over to make sure we were all right, and every single one of them wanted to stay there with us, offering to let us wait in the warmth of their cars. We were grateful, but Mike had already called someone from work to come get us, and surely the police would be there momentarily.

Still, we were touched at the sincerity of every offer, and it didn't escape either of us that had this happened in a few other places we had been stationed, the only people who would have stopped would have done so in order to see what we had in the truck that would be worth their time to get out of their car and grab. In the roughly six months we had been in North Dakota we'd begun to learn about the generosity of its people and about their collective inherent kindness. We had no doubts that we could have taken any one of those people up on their offers of warmth and dry refuge, and we would have been fine.

NoDaks (as North Dakotans sometimes fondly call themselves) are hearty, kind people. They take care of each other. If not for the long, hard winters, it's a place we could have easily called home after retirement from the USAF.

But at that moment, I despised the snow. The snow I had wanted so badly. We'd *wrecked* because of it. The truck we had *just* paid off was toast, and we didn't have another car to fall back on.

We were kind of screwed.

But we were all right. We walked away from that wreck without a scratch on either of us, and we were positive that we were all right.

~

Life without a car during the winter was not the torture we thought it would be. We lived on the air force base, and everything we absolutely needed was within two miles; we could walk to the commissary and drag a duffle bag along (and invariably on the way out someone we knew would be there, and would offer a ride home), we could walk to the base theater for a cheap second-release movie, we had the BX and its plethora of Soccer Mom designer duds with a Burger King in the same building, and across the street was the bowling alley.

We were stuck on base, but we weren't *stuck*.

One week after the accident, Mike was paged to come into work; as a Certified Registered Nurse Anesthetist, when an emergency calls, he has to answer. There was little risk of being needed to provide anesthesia for a trauma; those cases were routinely sent into Grand Forks to the hospital there, but there were emergencies now and then. Women going into labor often wanted epidurals, and they loved Mike and his drugs. When the call to work came—some heavily pregnant woman wanted to fall in love with his magical fun drugs— we were at the bowling alley for Friday Night League play; he finished up his game quickly, and left. The base hospital was less than a block away, and he could cut across the BX parking lot to get there.

It would take him less than five minutes. Cross the street, cross the BX parking lot, and bingo, there's the side door to the base's it's-not-a-clinic-it's-a-tiny-hospital. Not a problem.

Fifteen minutes later I was paged to the bowling alley's phone.

"Umm," was the first thing I heard after picking up the receiver.

Umm.

In his hurry to get to the hospital to pump happy fun drugs into the laboring woman, Mike slipped and fell in the ice-covered BX parking lot and broke his ankle. He heard it pop; after a moment of consideration ("Well...hell.") he pulled himself up and hobbled the rest of the way, but there was no denying that he had become the patient instead of the care provider.

His partner was called in to cover the epidural while Mike was taken into Grand Forks to have an orthopedist look at his x-rays to confirm that yep, that sucker was broken.

I wanted to know why he had gotten up and walked from the parking lot to the hospital when he had a giant brick of a cell phone in his pocket and could have called for help, but that's really neither here nor there. I just have a need to point it out at every opportunity.

So now it's winter in North Dakota, we have no car, and Mike's on crutches.

It started to feel as if we really were a little bit stuck.

I could still walk to the commissary and BX for food and anything else we needed, or I could send the teenager, but Mike had a slight issue. Busted ankle or not, he still had to show up for work, even though he wasn't allowed to do anesthesia. I wasn't sure how he was going to get there, but he still had to report as normal every morning, where he would then spend the day rolling around the hospital in a wheelchair, doing paperwork and anything else they could find to keep him busy.

I was beginning to think I would have to walk to the BX to buy a sled and then drag his sorry ass to the hospital every day.

We caught a break when a friend offered the use of his Bronco for as long as we needed it. His family had two vehicles and only one driver, so it wasn't going to be missed.

Relief.

We were no longer stuck on base; soon after that we were able to plunk down a thousand bucks as a down payment on another car, and we were on our way.

Life was getting back to normal.

North Dakota Normal.

~

A few weeks later, I began having a nagging pain in my left hip. It wasn't horrible, but it wasn't going away, either. Someone with a voodoo doll had probably grabbed a nice sized needle and shoved it into the buttocks of a nice fuzzy Thumper doll, aiming straight for the hip joint. Or I was simply overweight and out of shape, and if I would get off my asterisk and exercise, it would hurt less.

Being the intelligent person that I am, I decided to ignore it. I waited for whatever sick person playing with the voodoo doll to pull the stick out of my ass.

After all, it was only achy; it wasn't excruciating and the pain rarely made me limp.

I could live with it. That certainly seemed easier than going to the gym.

~

Part of living in an area where harsh winter is the norm is preparing for the inevitabilities of what tends to happen during said harsh winters. You stockpile ready-to-eat food and have plenty of warm clothing on hand; you have an alternate heat source, and develop a plan about what you will do during a catastrophic weather event.

As our first winter approached we had every intention of assembling an emergency kit, complete with food we wouldn't need to cook and candles for light and warmth. If we could squeeze it out of the budget, we might even add a small propane stove or heater to the kit. Our intentions were admirable.

The pathway to Hell, and all that.

With every blizzard that hit, we mumbled to ourselves about the need for those emergency supplies, but never actually did anything about it. And we didn't need them; as winter trailed off into spring we'd never lost power for more than a few hours, and we were all capable of going those few hours without hot food. We had blankets and sweatpants; we could even keep the dog warm.

We were rock stars. We had the whole living in North Dakota thing nailed down.

In early April 1997, when the first hints of spring would have been most welcome and were certainly expected, the state was hit with major winter weather; it began with freezing rain and rapidly escalated into pounding wind and snow. The initial frozen rain wrapped itself neatly around power lines, and as the rain turned to heavy, wet snow, the weight of ice and snow being whipped by blizzard-force winds cracked utility poles, sending them down like dominos.

It wasn't just the air force base; Highway 2 was closed across the state, and people gritted their teeth against it, praying that no one would die in this last-blast-of-the-season blizzard.

It sucked; it was cold and wet, but the only thing people collectively wanted was for everyone to come through it all right. That was the mantra on the radio: let's all make it out alive. And we almost made it; there were two fatalities, a woman and her child, having gone off a road into a creek, managed to get out of their car and headed for a nearby house, only to succumb to the cold before they could get there.

That was a sobering, heart-wrenching wake-up call. Winter could be a real bitch.

The power was out for four days, and because of the bitter cold that seeped through the triple paned windows, we slept in the basement—the warmest part of the house—on the floor. We dragged Curt's twin bed mattress down from the second story for him and we used the thin mattress from a sleeper-sofa. Our only heat came from a thick votive candle – one we had to borrow from a neighbor, because our emergency kit was still in the planning stages. The cold permeated the house horrifically, and within a day the dog was groggy and there was ice floating in the toilets.

We didn't worry about it, other than the dog who inexplicably refused to go down the stairs into the basement; we knew it wasn't going to last. Where we were not prepared, the base was, and there was warmth to be found at the gym; they had generator power and we could go there for an hour or two, and we could even grab a hot meal in the transient mess hall set up on the basketball court. Life was uncomfortable but not problematic; sooner or later power would be restored, we would again have heat, and everything would be fine.

On the fourth night, as we rolled into day five of post-blizzard wonder, the power kicked back on and with it the furnace came to life, and by morning we were all nice and toasty.

The dog was all right.

My hip hurt significantly more, but I'd just spent four nights sleeping on a very thin mattress on a cold basement floor. Of course things were going to hurt.

That was just normal.

And hey, we'd survived what surely had to be the worst of what North Dakota weather could shovel out.

Things were just going to get better.

Right?

~

Two weeks later, Spring gripped Grand Forks like a five year old holding a squirming puppy. The temperature shot up, the snow melted, and the Red River rose. There were feverish but well coordinated sand bagging efforts; most of the town showed up at various locations to fill and place sandbags. Buses shuttled base residents into town so that military members and their families could help. People shoveled sand until their hands blistered and bled, and they wired shut bags until their fingers were red and raw. Lines formed along the levy and bags were stacked one after the other, hope held in tight breaths that the effort would be enough.

The river rose quickly, and in spite of the incredible efforts of Grand Forks' citizens sand bagging to a height well over what the predicted flood level would be, the river rose higher, a break formed in the levy, and the city was flooded. Homes were swallowed by the crushing tide of water that poured from the river; downtown Grand Forks was mostly under water and—oddly—on fire, and the order to evacuate was issued.

As people fled the city, the air force base prepared to receive the masses. A hangar was converted into a shelter, with an endless sea of cots. Residents of the base did what they could, gathering clothing, taking in pets. School was canceled, because the on-base elementary and middle schools were needed as emergency medical centers, being quickly converted into nursing homes and urgent care offices. The stress level on base was high, but controlled.

I counted myself lucky, and wondered why my left foot was now hurting every bit as much as my hip.

~

Because I am so intelligent, in the midst of hip and foot pain, I decided to take up golf. It was a ballet of horror; I had a wicked slice, my form was terrible, and I couldn't hit the ball more than a hundred yards. Nine holes of golf yielded for me a score of around 120 and toddleresque frustration. So of course my back and shoulders began to hurt; I was doing something physically unfamiliar, and I'd get used to it eventually. My form would improve and along with it my score, and all the walking was good for me. I was having fun and loved it, so the achiness wasn't a problem.

Right?

I slogged my way through the rest of spring and part of summer, cursing the unfairness of only being in my thirties with my body already falling apart. There wasn't much on me that didn't hurt and over the counter pain relievers did nothing for it, but it wasn't *that* bad, so why bother a doctor about it?

So my hip ached. No big deal. So what if my foot had joined it, along with a chorus formed by my back, shoulders, and other hip? My knee was beginning to sing soprano, bellowing above the rest of the chorus in an effort to be heard. I blew it all off as residual damage drilled into my body from a couple of years of competition-level TaeKwonDo—even though it had been at least seven years since I had competed—and decided that adding bowling (at which I was fairly good) and golf (at which I was not) into the mix was my problem.

It would get better.

It had to get better.

As mosquito-season started to wane into Almost Winter, I caved. I went to see a doctor on base, and to my complete non-surprise, he couldn't find anything wrong.

But, he believed that I was in pain and had been.

Later, that would be something I would appreciate.

He ordered blood work that came back normal, sent me to physical therapy that didn't work, then ran more blood work to check for Lyme Disease. When that also came back normal, he began to poke at odd places on my body.

He asked question after question; most of them he had asked before, but this felt different. He was looking for something new, some thread he wanted to tie together. How long had I been in pain? Where and when did it begin? Had I felt it in all four quadrants of my body? Did over-the-counter pain medications even begin to touch it? Was it preceded by a traumatic event?

He poked some more.

That hurt like hell.

"I think," he said almost carefully, weighing my reaction, "that you have Fibromyalgia."

Fibrowhahootia?

"I want to send you to a rheumatologist for confirmation."

Well, wonderful. Let's send the person who hates going to the doctor to another doctor. That will be so much fun.

The rheumatologist, a five feet three inch tall fellow who weighed in at about three hundred fifty pounds, proclaimed me to be an obese white female with pleasantly warm hands and oddly cold legs, took a lengthy history, poked at me again, and agreed with my air force doctor.

Fibromyalgia.

But, on the bright side, he said it would run its course in about nine months. I'd be fine if I just waited it out.

I'd been researching the disease online, working hard to separate the facts from the freaked out postings by people who were living with the disease, and it took major effort to not cough *bullshit* into my hand.

I didn't know a lot about it, but I did know three things: most doctors considered it to be a wastebasket diagnosis designed to shut problematic patients up, it was never going away, and it wasn't going to kill me.

That latter thing? After some of what I'd read, I wasn't sure that was a good thing.

~

Over the next two years, I didn't get any better, but I didn't get any worse, either. I had other aches and pains that were obviously not related to having FMS and I had them checked out, just in case. By early 1999 I had an additional diagnosis of Chronic Myofasical Pain Syndrome, but to me it was just another way of saying "now everything hurts."

19

Rather than the undefined muscle pain of FMS, the CMPS was fairly clear in that it was pain felt in the outer lining of the muscles.

There was no cure for that, either.

Still, it wasn't too bad. I still bowled halfway decently. I still golfed horribly. I was doing getting by.

I was doing fine.

Until I wasn't.

By March 1999 my legs discovered whole new levels of pain; my quads were gripped in a vise-like fist of fire that changed my gait and killed my knees and I walked in old-lady shuffles, hunched over to keep my balance. By mid-April, Mike checked out a wheelchair from the hospital, because it was the only way I was getting out of the house.

There was no more golfing.

No more bowling.

No walking to the BX for the hell of it.

We lived in a two-story duplex; the stairs were so challenging that I avoided them. I went downstairs in the morning to let the dog out, grab food, and then went upstairs until someone else was home. I would have avoided the trip upstairs if we'd had a bathroom downstairs. I sat at my desk in the spare bedroom and tried to write, but most of the time I couldn't concentrate enough to cough up anything coherent. I surfed around Prodigy—what being online meant at the time—and chatted with friends, and I played a lot of computer solitaire.

I moved as little as possible, because when I did, the ugly happened. My face contorted, I sucked in breath in odd little gasps, and it looked all too phony.

The more real it felt, the more I felt like it looked to other people like I was exaggerating.

In June we found ourselves packing up to move again, because the USAF had decided it was time for another permanent change of station. The base hospital was being downgraded to clinic status, and Mike's services as an anesthesia provider would no longer be needed there.

We didn't mind, because this move was taking us back to California. To home.

Surely things there would be perfectly all right.

Right?

~

Within four months of returning to California, the pain in my legs abated enough that I was back on my feet. It was a small victory; I enjoyed not having to get around in a wheelchair, especially not having my face at everyone else's ass-height.

People, a lot of you? Not quite hygienic enough.

It wasn't a perfect return to mobile glory, though. I lost quite a bit of lean muscle mass, which left me flabbier than before, and instead of specific pain—my hip, my foot, my legs—everything hurt, and it hurt pretty much all the time. From the time I got up in the morning until I went to bed, I ached much like you do the first couple of days just after a new exercise routine: uncomfortable, but not worth whining about.

The sad thing about having pain like that is that you get used to it. While I didn't have to stop and think, "Oh yeah, that hurts," I also wasn't curled up in a tight little ball because the pain was that bad. It wasn't. It was persistent but not incapacitating, so I gradually started getting back to Real Life.

If you asked me how bad it was, I probably shrugged it off with, "Eh, not too bad," even on the days when it was That Bad.

I understood something very fundamental: no one wants to hear about someone else's pain all the time. It doesn't matter if it's wrapped around you and chafing like sandpaper

21

drawn across soft skin; other people get tired of hearing about it. They can't fix it, they can't fix you, so after a while mentioning it just becomes whining static; you're either an attention seeking freak (because no one can be in *that* much pain *that* often and still be coherent, right?) or you get tuned out.

I don't blame anyone for that.

I don't want to hear about someone else's never ending stream of complaints either.

Part of the return to Real Life was finishing that novel that had been languishing in the bottom of a box for years; I'd been editing a martial arts e-zine and had attracted some editorial attention, and was highly encouraged to finish it and polish it. As I zeroed in on my creative juices, I found I cared less and less about the aches and pains that plagued me.

Still hurt, sure, but so what? I was *doing*. And as long as I was doing, I wanted to expand my horizons a bit; I went back to college.

In August 2001 I headed back to school, taking Spanish, a class in using Pagemaker publishing software, and—even I was surprised—body conditioning.

I turned 40 that August. I was tired of being fat and flabby along with being in pain, and since the pain wasn't going anywhere and the P.E. class was there and dirt cheap, I decided to go for it. After all, it couldn't hurt any worse, right?

On the first morning after the first conditioning class, I invented several new and colorful swear words. Getting out of bed damn near required vodka and a crow bar. I moved like a ninety year old woman who'd had one foot amputated and the other smashed with a hammer.

It wasn't pretty.

It also wasn't permanent. I knew it wasn't going to be permanent. That made it tolerable.

After a couple of weeks I felt stronger and I was a couple of pounds lighter. I could say, "My name is Karen" in Spanish and I could open Pagemaker on a computer without wondering what damage I was going to inflict on the hard drive. By the time the semester was nearing its end, I was actually managing a very slow jog around the school's track; I'd only dropped six pounds, but knowing that I survived the class and had likely put on a little muscle, that made the disappointing poundage fine.

I registered for the next semester, quite happy with the idea of making further strides.

Life was good.

~

Four days after Christmas, a treasured friend died. I'm still not sure what happened, but it began when she fell off a toilet. She also had Fibromyalgia, but was also saddled with Lupus and was a newly diagnosed diabetic, rendering her medical treatment a bit more complicated than the average Jane's, but no one could have seen the turns she would take. She began losing her vision, and said in an email that she felt so bad that it felt like she was dying.

I took that to mean, "Yo, I really feel like crap. Really bad. Really really bad."

I didn't think it meant she actually thought she was dying.

I blew it off and told her she wasn't allowed to die.

In November, she went into the hospital. For whatever reasons, she was transferred to another hospital and her complete records didn't go with her: she wasn't being given her insulin.

She wound up in ICU.

One by one, her organs began to fail.

And then in a gut punch to everyone who loved her, she died.

I lost any drive to go back to school after the semester break. I decided that because my book had just come out and I was plodding through another, that it might be better to skip Spanish 2 and P.E. and just work. After all, I had the Spanish textbook and could pick my way through it, and the air force base we were living on had a great gym; I only needed some self-discipline and I could get the book done, learn a little more Spanish, and work out.

Stop laughing.

I made steady progress on the book, worked out a little, and was feeling pretty good. Menopause was rearing its ugly head a little early, but I wasn't having hot flashes. In fact, as far as I could tell I was experiencing the world's easiest menopause. One month everything was normal, the next – my body seemed to have edited out its personal punctuation.

Worry over it? Why? I was forty years old. If it wasn't menopause, then it was surely peri-menopause. I might have another period in a month or two, or the hot flashes might begin. The idea of getting older sucked, but the idea of no more dealing with cramps and the like?

Sign me up.

I admit, when the semester started I began to wish I had sucked it up and gone, but the book was coming along and I was having a good time writing it, and it seemed like everything was as on track as it had ever been.

Then came a phone call; my mother had a large, odd lump, underwent a biopsy, and the result: it was malignant, and it was lymphoma. While she underwent chemo and radiation, I decided to push myself to get the book done as soon as possible.

Just in case.

She'd liked the first book, so…just in case.

I spent my days planted at my desk, typing away; the story was in my head already, it was simply a matter of getting it out and onto virtual paper. I sat there and typed, got up to pee, went to the kitchen for a drink, then back to my desk.

At some point it occurred to me that I was taking an awful lot of breaks just to pee.

And I was drinking an awful lot.

When the dog began to sigh in resignation every time I stepped over him to get to the bathroom, I mentioned it to Mike; he's a nurse, he would know if my escalating thirst and urination had gone from being the byproduct of a diet soda addiction to something more insidious. We both started paying more attention to the sheer volume of liquids I was pouring down my throat and the number of subsequent trips to the bathroom.

It was during a routine trip to Walmart that the scales tipped from "maybe this is a problem" to "oh, hell, this is a problem." I'd mentioned being thirsty once or twice already, but as we passed the fish tanks in the pet department, I contemplated sticking my head in one and sucking it dry.

Once we were out of the store I headed straight for a vending machine and bought a can of iced tea, drained it, and bought another.

We were both thinking it: diabetes.

He called the appointment line at the base hospital to see how quickly I could get in to see our doctor; the technician on the other end determined that I surely wasn't drinking *that* much, so it wasn't an emergency. I could have an appointment in two weeks.

Two very long weeks.

My thirst had reached epic proportions; Mike stood in line at KFC one afternoon and I sat at a table, waiting, twitching like a junkie waiting for a fix, staring at the soda fountain and thinking that I could just go stick my head under a nozzle and turn it on. In the ten minutes it took him to get through line and place an order I went from being really thirsty to *Oh holy hell this hurts*.

I didn't even put ice in the cup; that would just take up precious space where liquid could be.

I was Gollum with Diet Mountain Dew.

My precious...

By the time I first saw a doctor it was early May; Mike went with me (partly for support, partly for information, and a whole lot of making sure I actually showed up for the appointment) and we both assumed it was going to be a matter of getting some blood work, finding out my glucose was too high, then having more blood work done, after which I would hop onto the diabetic hamster wheel and start running. We envisioned some hefty life changes: diet, exercise, tricky medication timing, all doable.

Just for kicks, I mentioned to the doc that while my primary complaints were excessive thirst and urination, I also hadn't had a period since early January. But you know, being forty and all...

I should have worried when that slice of news seemed to give him pause. But, he did as we expected; he ordered up blood work and sent me home. A few days later Mike accessed my lab file on the hospital computer and printed the results out – my blood glucose was 95.

Perfectly normal.

So what, then?

The next day the doc called; yes, my blood glucose was normal but my prolactin levels were elevated. It wasn't by a lot, but enough to concern him. It explained the amenorrhea—my missing personal punctuation—as well as the marathon drinking and peeing. The only hitch in all that?

If it was what he suspected, there was a tumor on my pituitary gland.

You know.

A brain tumor.

~

No one asked me if I wanted a ride on the medical merry-go-round, but I suddenly found myself with a fistful of tickets and no way out of the short line that moved far too quickly toward it. I wanted to be on the roller coaster instead; make my way through the long, slow moving line, hop on for a too-short thrill, and then get off with the relief of *that was kind of cool* amusement.

My primary care doctor was sharp; he put the pieces together based on the symptoms and lab results alone, but he needed an MRI to confirm his suspicions. I'd had MRIs done on my knee before; that was going to be a 6-8 week wait, which would give me nearly two months of not knowing as well as nearly two months of plausible denial.

It would fix itself while I waited for my time in the tube.

Surely it would.

The problem with the direction my brain was going was that I hadn't considered the triage aspect of assigning appointments for the MRI machine. I had to wait to have my knee peeked at because it wasn't exactly important. And apparently, even the USAF medical machine considers a potential brain tumor to be fairly important.

A day after I talked to my doctor, the radiology clinic called with my appointment date. Instead of having weeks to mentally prepare myself, I had one day. The call came in around 2 p.m. and they had a slot for me at 10:30 p.m. the next day.

Wisely, Mike called my doctor and told him that Valium would be a good idea; I'd handled the confines of the MRI when my knee was being examined, but this time I would be going in head-first and there was more riding on the results than whether or not I would have to give up TaeKwonDo for awhile.

By this point, we hadn't told anyone what was going on; my mother was being treated for lymphoma and we didn't want to worry her over what could be nothing. And until we had something more than a Maybe, we didn't want to tell our son anything. He was 18 and old enough to shoulder some uncertainty, but why give it to him until we had to?

With the doctor's presumed diagnosis and a firm appointment for the MRI, it was time to let him know what was going on. He was in his room at his desk, and I had just gotten off the phone with the radiology clinic; I was headed down the hall but not specifically to tell him anything, but when I saw him there, I knew that was the time.

After all, it was probably "just" a pituitary tumor I was looking at. Nothing to really worry about.

So I stopped and lingered at his bedroom door, and tried to casually tell him I was having an MRI done the next night. I fully intended to tell him without any drama, to drive home the point that it was no big deal.

I told him about the MRI, but when it came to the reason why I needed one, every intention I had crumbled and my voice caught; I managed to choke out that I "might have a tumor" and pointed to my head.

Until that moment, I hadn't been scared.

My 18 year old son got up and crossed the room in two long strides and had his arms around me before I could completely fall apart.

~

Okay... so I had this thing growing in my head. Initially I thought I was in menopause (and relished the idea), but in late March or early April 2002 I realized I was drinking an awful lot; it sort of crept up on me, varying degrees of thirst day after day, until I realized one morning that I was sucking down at least 64 ounces of anything cold and fluid I could get my hands on first thing every morning, and I kept drinking in massive quantities all day long. The end result of drinking so much is...well, you know.

What I didn't realize is the…well, you know…was causing the incredible thirst. Being so thirsty all the time spurred the Spouse Thingy into making me an appointment with our primary care doctor at Travis AFB; he thought I might be diabetic.

The doc agreed with him; this was something that needed to be looked into. He made note of the fact that I was pretty sure I was in the throes of menopause and ordered a shitload of blood work to be done. The vampires at the lab surely loved this; they sucked out at least 5 tubes of blood and made me pee in this tiny, tiny cup (ok, a Big Gulp cup is tiny when you're drinking 3 gallons a day.)

My blood sugar came back at 95. Perfectly normal.

My prolactin level, however, came back at 118. Normal is less than 10.

And then there was this merry go round of drinking and peeing.

("What did you do today?" "I peed.")

Something was amiss. My doc, being fairly sharp, caught the implications right off the bat. The likely culprit to my problems was a pituitary tumor. He ordered an MRI—and I complied, as much as I didn't want to—and the evidence was right there. Glaring bright white against the black film of the MRI.

I had a tumor.

A brain tumor.

And it was big.

The MRI immediately went to the base hospital's neurosurgeon; she looked and measured, checked my lab values, looked some more, and decided this was an Unusual Tumor, unusual enough that she didn't want to handle it. She wanted me to see a civilian pituitary specialist. Someone who could look at the MRI and have a better idea what it might be. Someone who wouldn't just be using me for the value of experience. Between her efforts and the efforts of my primary care doc, and numerous inquiries by the Spouse Thingy, I got an appointment—fairly quickly, too—with a civilian specialist.

He took one look at the MRI and was brutally honest. He couldn't tell exactly what it was, either. It appeared to be cystic in nature, but it was not the ordinary pituitary adenoma, and it was creeping up the pituitary stalk toward my hypothalamus. The only way to know for sure was to take it out.

Take it out.

Of my *brain*.

Holy shit.

~

I did a lot of reading about pituitary tumors while I waited for this appointment; I knew how he would take it out (go in under the upper lip, drill through the sinuses to get to the pituitary gland, yank that sucker out, pack my sinuses, close up, no visible scar), and I knew that the surgery itself was becoming almost routine. But this was MY brain. My pituitary gland. My tumor.

I was terrified.

In between that visit and the day of surgery, I had every possible ill outcome running through my head, the least of which was the chance that I could come out of this blind—the optic nerve runs far too close to the pituitary for my taste. So do the carotid arteries. More than anything I wanted a feeling of serenity about this, some sign that it would be all right. Some sign that I wasn't seeing things for the last time. Something to tell me I would see my son's face again, see my husband, even see the cat lick himself inappropriately and the dog eat his own poop. Something to tell me that my last breath was not going to be drawn on an operating table.

Over the three weeks between seeing the neurosurgeon

and the scheduled surgery, people with pituitary tumors seemed to be coming out of the woodwork. They popped up in email, in casual conversations. Invariably, they had the same message. "I have one. I had one. I'm doing fine."

They were comforting, but this was still My Brain Tumor, and inside I was shaking like the proverbial leaf.

Two days before the surgery The Spouse Thingy and I had dinner at the BX food court. Normally we didn't get the Chinese food there—it wasn't the greatest—but on this night the lines for everything else were long and we didn't want to wait, so we settled for it. Each dinner came with a fortune cookie; I never eat mine, I always give them to him. Like always, he shoved it towards me and told me I had to at least open it myself.

He read his; it was typical fortune cookie nonsense. Scratch your palm and blink twice and all life's richest will come your way.

I read mine: *You will live a long and happy life.*

I wanted to cry. It felt like the sign I'd been—literally—praying for.

~

The next day was dedicated to pre-operative appointments: getting a chest x-ray, more blood drawn, an EKG. As part of that appointment merry-go-round I was also given my scheduled surgery time.

First case of the day.

Be at the hospital at 5:30 a.m.

The hospital, UCD Medical Center, is in Sacramento. We lived 50 miles away, at Travis AFB, which meant that we'd have to get up by 4 a.m. and be out on the road before 4:30. In the fricking morning!

Did I mention I am not a morning person?

I took my pillow with me and snoozed on the ride up

there (as opposed to puking up my toenails the entire way, which is what I was sure I'd be doing.) We checked in at 5:30, whereupon they handed me this thin, tiny gown designed to allow me to moon the entire hospital, stuck us in a room where we waited for at least an hour for an OR escort (not as kinky as it sounds.) I expected to be hurling large chunks across the room, but didn't.

By this point I think I was resigned to the idea that there was no escape. They had my clothes; where was I going to go with my backside shining like a bright white beacon off the shores of the California coast? They had me. I was doomed.

The OR escort finally arrived; I was put on a gurney and taken up to the recovery room, where Mike introduced me to the Certified Registered Nurse Anesthetist he had hand-picked to knock me out and keep me knocked through the surgery. Nick (said CRNA) carefully explained what he would be doing to me, including all the things I would never remember, and then stuck an IV in my hand. While I laid there, contemplating the dark, dreary recovery room, the neurosurgeon (Mike hand picked him, too) popped in to say hello (and promised, no, I won't sneeze while I have my fingers in your brain); Nick gave me something through the IV (Versed, I think), and I was off to LaLa Land. I felt all warm and fuzzy…and then nothing.

Next thing I knew I was in the recovery room with someone sitting at my side (recovery room nurse, male, that's all I know) who was urging me to breathe. *Deep breaths. More. That's good.* Mike appeared at various points (I should point out that he moonlighted at UCDMC and was allowed where family members normally are not); I recall hearing the nurse tell him that I'd been given morphine and my breathing rate was depressed, at 8-10 per minute.

My brain interpreted that as "She stopped breathing."

After about three hours (or so I'm told; it could have been ten minutes or ten hours as far as I was concerned) I was finally taken to my room. I was transferred to a bed, and while lying there half out of my drugged head, I heard him.

The Yeller.

I couldn't tell exactly where he was on the floor; I could only hear his booming voice echoing through the hallways. *HELP ME HELP ME! WHERE'S MY DOCTOR? I WANT TO GO!*

I was thinking, "Oh shut the fark up," but all I could do was concentrate on breathing.

HELP ME!

Gawwwddd…

At some point—it felt like minutes later but could have been hours—a nurse placed these THINGS on my legs. White THINGS with Velcro straps. Mike told me they were to massage my legs, and to keep me from developing blood clots.

My intelligent response: "Noooooooooooo."

Later he told me I was getting a roommate. "Nooooooooooo."

I whined a lot.

~

Mike stayed until at least 11:30 that night; he made sure that I could reach my water, kept my pitcher full and stayed until he was sure that I could get the cup on my own, refill it using the pitcher on the table, and call for a nurse to bring more water when I needed it. The water was critical; the tumor had caused a condition called *Diabetes Insipidus* (the short of it: my body no longer made the natural anti-diuretic hormone, Vasopressin, causing my kidneys to just let water flow through with no stops; I had a medication for it but they weren't giving it to me so they could see what would happen… at some point what happened was a burst collection bag and massive amounts of urine all over the floor) and I needed to be able to input as much as I output (all hail the mighty catheter!) He had gotten nine pitchers of water for me throughout the day; that night I drank six more.

I was more coherent the next day; so was The Yeller. At some point he must have been sedated, but I awoke to strains of *LET ME OUT! HELP!* over and over.

Mike appeared early, followed shortly by the Physical Therapist Lady. They sat me up at the side of the bed, and then helped me stand; I was on my feet for only about half a minute, which garnered me praise worthy of an Oscar Nominee (or at least a Gold Star), but it left me with the Headache from Hell.

The nurse said she would get me morphine for the pain; by this point I was half out of it and started crying, telling Mike "Noooooooooo, I don't want to stop breathing..." He tried to assure me it would be fine, my breathing rate might slow a little bit, but I kept whining, "I don't want to stop breathing."

Okay.

I was terrified, really.

They gave me the morphine in spite of my whining reservations and I was determined to not fall back asleep; I was going to stay awake and BREATHE. Deep breaths. Numerous breaths. I would inhale as if I were trying to suck up the mother of all lines.

I was going to breathe so well that I would win the Golden Lung award.

Right around lunchtime both Curt and Mike's parents showed up; they found me sitting up in bed, a bowl of Jello in hand, and fast asleep. When I did stir, I proclaimed that the Jello sucked, then went back to sleep, periodically waking up with a start, forcing myself to breathe.

Nope, I would not let the morphine do me in. I was going to breathe.

(Yes, all right, hindsight tells me that if I was waking up,

I was breathing all along, but dammit, I was being proactive!
I was breathing!)

When late afternoon came Mike said he needed to get home early because Curt had to work and couldn't feed the animals or let the dog out to pee. My mature reaction?

"Nooooooo. I don't want to be alone."

So, being the good Spouse Thingy that he is, he stayed a little longer and talked to my roommate's husband some.

This would be Mumbling Mary. She'd had a disk fusion, Herrington rods inserted to stabilize her spine, and a nerve in her leg worked on. She was in some serious pain. They started her out with a boatload of narcotics, but they were giving her less than what she normally took just to survive the pain. She was four-years post-major-car-accident and existed on Percoset and Other Fun Drugs. A pain management team finally stopped by to assess her, doubled the amount of drugs that she was getting, and that second day she finally got some rest.

This was a good thing for Mary, but it totally screwed up her sense of day and night and left her high as a kite. That third day I was fairly coherent, sitting up, even walked the hall some (and got my nasal packing out – giant tampons they'd shoved into my sinuses), and she slept through most of it, occasionally waking to tell her husband to fix the clock already; she determined that it said 3:30 and she *knew* it was 8:30 (it was 1 p.m.) Around 9 p.m., just as I was falling asleep, she decided it was daytime. The nurses came in to turn her (an exercise in agony for poor Mumbling Mary) and she wanted to know where her husband was; they tried to explain that it was night time and he'd gone home, but she was sure they were lying. He couldn't have gone home – he hadn't fixed the clock!

I was *almost* asleep when The Yeller started back up. He was also throwing things, creating a general atmosphere of unpleasantness and construction zone noise, and I was finally able to determine that he was in the next room. He was screaming for the hospital administrator, calling his nurse 'Nurse Ratchet,' begging to leave, loudly declaring his want of going home. Mary, in the meantime, couldn't find her call button, so I pulled the curtain back and asked if she needed help. "Oh no, I just need to find this," and she was moving around so much I was afraid she'd hurt herself, so I buzzed the nurse from my bed.

~

After that Mary decided I was her best friend ever and proceeded to talk. And talk. And talk. The thing was, she wasn't really talking to me; she was carrying on conversations with the voices in her head. Around 4 a.m. she turned on her TV, and Wimbledon was playing. She muttered things like "Don't hit that tennis ball. You'll break the vase." She talked to everyone she knew, *all* night long.

It was too funny to be seriously annoying.

What was truly annoying was the blood they wanted to draw from me, every six hours around the clock. After the first two days the veins in my right arm pretty much shut down and because of the I.V. they couldn't take blood out of my left. My arms had track marks worthy of a junkie, but they were getting no blood. Needle after needle…the blood just would not flow. I was bruised, sore, and still they wanted more.

Late on the third night, after trying for a third time to get more than a thimble's worth of blood out of me, the nurse declared that was it; she refused to torture me any more. I was stable, I'd been stable, she had no doubt I would continue to be stable, and if the doctors really wanted another late-night blood sample, they could send someone from the lab to get it.

It must not have been important enough, because I was

finally able to sleep for a long stretch without the light flicking on and someone telling me "just a little poke."

Saturday morning I woke up, felt great, walked the hall without the aid of a walker, then talked to an endocrinologist and a few of the surgical residents, who all deemed me fit to go home. I was alert and could walk unassisted, and recovery would go much faster at home.

No argument from me; at home I only needed to deal with a psychotic cat; I wouldn't have to listen to The Yeller threaten to jump off the bed into the toilet another time.

Once I was home I could sit in the living room and watch TV. Or I could sit at my desk and play online. It'd be fun.

The ride home completely wiped me out. I got home and went to bed, and for the most part stayed there for two more days. The fatigue clung to me for almost a week. So did the swollen face. Initially I looked like I'd gone a round or two with Mike Tyson; after a few days I only looked like a TeleTubby.

Tinky Winky.

I had survived. The surgeon didn't sneeze with his fingers in my brain. I didn't go blind. He got it all. From that point all we could do was to wait for the pathology report, and hope that I wasn't one of the Very Rare People to get pituitary cancer.

~

I wasn't.

I am one of the very *very* Rare People to get *lymphocytic hypophysitis.* Very rare.

Extremely rare.

Extremely lucky.

It's Latin that basically means I had a giant zit-like mass in my brain, and because I had the tumor removed, I'm cured. It probably won't come back.

It left me with a few issues; I'll have diabetes insipidus for the rest of my life and will have to pay close attention to how much I drink, how much I sweat, and if my weight skyrockets from one day to the next. I have issues with my cortisol levels. My brain no longer makes growth hormone, which means I have practically zero chance of gaining any lean muscle mass, and I'm flabbier because of it. It knocked out my thyroid. It exacerbated my reactive hypoglycemia.

But.

I got to live.

It was proof, after all, that I have a brain.

~

What the hell did I just do?

That was the thought that settled over my brain like an itchy blanket the moment after I registered to walk in the Susan G. Komen 3 Day for the Cure in San Francisco for 2010.

I had a laundry list of medical reasons to not even think of trying this. I spent an entire night mulling over those reasons, from the accident that seemed to be the trigger for Fibromyalgia to the lingering brain tumor issues. Taking on the training for this walk could, without exaggerating, be a bad idea.

Some risks are worth taking, if there are good enough reasons.

I had one reason to take the risk. Her name was Anne, and she was a long-distance friend of mine. We met online in a Fibromyalgia newsgroup and became friends in an email ring shared with several other people.

We had chronic pain in common, but then, too, while I was slogging through the brain tumor minefield, she was battling breast cancer.

Right around the same time I got the good news about

my tumor, she got good news about hers.

We'd both fought, and we'd both won.

Our respective diseases, gone. Vanished. *Hasta la vista, baby*.

She got the convertible I coveted before I did, but she deserved it.

When we were in North Dakota and the Spouse Thingy could not find the English teas that he loved, she sent him some. The Real Thing. From England. If he ran out, all I had to do was mention it, and the next day more was on the way.

Anne and I shared a birthday; I'd always taken a certain amount of joy in reminding her that regardless, she would always be several years older than I. I spent part of the week before our birthday in 2005 contemplating the e-card I was going to send her. Something appropriately insulting, but one sure to make her smile.

Four days before our birthday, I learned that she had died.

She was *fine*. They *said* she was fine. *They* said her cancer had not come back.

They were wrong.

I had reasons to not walk in a 3 Day event, but I had one very good one.

Her name was Anne, and I miss her.

The Places You'll Go. Or Not.
Just Wear Clean Socks.

"If you're going to walk, you need shoes," Murf said in an instant message.

I glanced at my feet; I was wearing shoes, thankyouverymuch, and they were fine shoes; bright white and barely scuffed at all. With my sensitive feet, I replaced my shoes on the average of every six months, so they were almost always new looking, and quite adequate to walk in. I said as much, and was met with a minute or two of online silence.

"You need the *right* shoes," he finally said. "Walking or more likely running shoes."

"I'm not *running* sixty freaking miles. I'm *walking*. And I have really good cross-trainers."

"You need walking or running shoes. And socks."

Socks?

Is he serious or is my leg being gently yanked upon?

"Go get fit for shoes," he insisted.

"My shoes fit."

He avoided calling me multiple names synonymous with "stubborn" and "stupid." The cross-trainers of which I was so fond, he explained, were all right for every day use (read: for sitting on your asterisk all day) but might not be ideal for training to walk long distances. They probably didn't flex enough, and undoubtedly didn't have enough room in the toe box to allow my foot to flatten properly.

Toe box?

Properly flattening feet?

WTF?

And *walking* socks?

"You want socks that will wick away sweat, and you want socks that won't cause friction. Sweat and friction cause blisters. Trust me."

Oh, I trusted him. I trusted my life-long friend so much that I engaged my Google-fu and began searching online for walking and running forums; either I'd find out that he was full of crap, or that I really did need magic shoes and socks.

~

I really needed magic shoes and socks.

After an evening of searching and reading different web sites, blogs, and forum posts, I realized that my Irish friend was not trying to pull one over on me; the consensus was clear: get professionally fit for the right shoes, and get the right socks.

"Body Glide," an experienced walker added to my list.

Fine.

"Blister bandages," someone else added. "Just in case."

I did another online search for shoe fitting, found a nearby store that offered such a service, and headed out.

~

"Take off your shoes and roll up your pants a bit," the sales guy told me after hearing what I was planning on doing. He was impressed by the endeavor, but not overly so; this was Fitness Boy, after all; he was obviously a runner and had likely heard it all from other chubby women coming in for new shoes. He didn't belittle the training in which I was about to engage, but he might not have believed it, either.

Face it, how many times do we all start some huge fitness thing and abandon it a week later? Treadmill clothes rack, anyone?

He had me walk to the other end of the store and back while he focused on my feet. I steeled myself to walk as normally as I could, but with someone judging my gait – it may not have been walking perfection.

"You have high, tight arches," he informed me after a cursory inspection of my feet. "That can cause a little hip pain..."

He had my attention.

He measured my feet, suggested orthotics for the high arches, and headed to the stockroom to select a few pairs of shoes for me to try.

Never once did the issue of price come up; apparently when one is looking for the right shoes, price is of no concern.

I decided that if the pair I wound up with rang up at $800, I would express concern.

Fitness Boy came back with three pairs of running shoes; you can walk in running shoes, he explained, but not run in walking shoes. And the running shoes have better flex in the toe box, which would allow my foot to flatten properly.

Bonus points for Murf.

I made a mental note of the price tags on the ends of each of the boxes, but while he was pulling shoes and lacing them I lost track of which were the least expensive and which might make me sob hysterically upon handing over my debit card. He handed me a pair of magic socks to wear while I was trying the shoes on, and I immediately noticed a difference in how they felt on my feet.

I dutifully tried on each pair and walked while he observed.

The first pair felt all right, but he noted a change in gait and pronation.

The second pair felt like I'd slipped gloves onto my feet; I was ready to scoop them up and run to the cash register, but he wanted me to try on the third pair, just in case.

Nope, it was the second pair.

My feet cried out in joy. Seriously. I could hear them weeping, *Finally*!

"They're high mileage shoes, around five hundred miles, but you'll want to come in about a month before your walk for a second pair so that you'll have time to break them in."

Ideally, he explained, I would want to alternate shoes during the walk, wearing one pair on days one and three, and the other pair the second day. That would give the shoes a chance to dry out and recover their flex over the day I wasn't wearing them.

Also, if my training took me into walking every day, I might want to buy a second pair earlier, to alternate every day.

I could do that.

I bought the shoes—which were actually the least expensive of the three—and the socks, and headed for home, a little nervous and a little excited, because in the morning I was taking my first training walk, and I was doing it in spiffy high mileage running shoes and magic socks.

* * * *

I am not a morning person. Morning for me doesn't begin until well after 9 a.m., and only then because the cats begin pestering me to get up and feed them. At nine, I'm pushing a furry paw off my face, or worse, a furry face away from my nose as Max tries to shove his entire self up one of my nostrils.

On the first day of training, though, I dragged myself up an hour early so that I could be out the door by nine, early enough to beat the heat. There was much moaning and under-my-breath cursing, but I got up, got dressed, confused the kitties, forced myself to eat breakfast, and was out the door a little before nine.

I had three miles planned, and had no idea how long that was going to take me.

That's 4.8 kilometers – which actually sounds worse than three miles, and now I wish it hadn't occurred to me.

In my brain it might as well have been thirty. I had visions of getting a mile away from home and having to sit down on a curb, out of breath and in pain, sweat pouring like tears of frustration off my body. I worried about nausea—would that first mile make me want to puke up my toenails?—but worse, I worried about massive digestive disturbances.

You can barf in the street. The other, not so much.

Somewhere around mile two I realized that I wasn't in much pain at all. I was beginning to have some hip achiness, but it wasn't the deep, OMG pain I was used to and had expected. It was surface pain, tight IT bands most likely, and not enough to make me want to sit down and give up. I kept walking, enjoying the nice wide sidewalks and bike paths that our little town has to offer, and hit the front door at 10 a.m.

Three miles in an hour. A perfectly acceptable pace.

Plus, I did not die.

That's always a bonus.

Surely my second day of walking would be just as successful; 3 mph isn't half bad for a beginner, and an hour out of my morning – that was nothing.

Enter the heat.

Day two required getting up at nearly seven in the morning to beat the early summer heat, which only confused the cats even more. Max greeted me with a look that was like, "Well, I'm not actually hungry, but you're up, so I'm required to start pestering you," and Buddah just stared at me like he was seeing feline royalty descend from the sky.

The hip pain held off until mile 2.5, but my feet were sweaty and sliding around in my shoes, making me question the magic socks. How magic can they be if I feel like I'm walking in a pool of slippery goo?

I made a mental note to look online for other magic sock options, wondering if I was going to regret buying three pairs of $10 socks.

Day two's three miles took a little over an hour; I wasn't happy, but hey, I was still a beginner. I'd get faster.

I sure as heck didn't see how I could get any slower.

~

Day three: five miles.

I played that over in my head the night before: five miles, five miles, five miles. I don't think I'd ever walked five miles at once, at least not intentionally. I might have a few times in high school before my friends and I started driving and co-opted our parents' cars, but that was probably also limited to walking around Marriot's Great America and punctuated with stops every 100 feet to get on the next ride.

I mapped out my route; I would head toward Burger King, a mile and a half away, where I would stop to make use of the facilities and grab an orange juice. Then I would walk down Pitt School Road, another mile. Turn around and go back, head towards home, and loop around the little park near the house until I was close to five miles

Piece o'cake.

Not being a morning person and certainly not one normally on foot, I didn't realize that on Saturday mornings Pitt School Road is busy, and after a few minutes of choking on car exhaust, I wanted to be somewhere else. So I turned down H Street and headed in a new direction, and wound up at one of the town's bigger parks.

I'd never noticed this park before.

This was Walker Nirvana.

The path around it was nearly a mile long—a tad over eight-tenths of a mile—and there were paths cutting through the park, it was tree-lined with stretches of shade, and best yet, there were two restrooms.

What more could a newby walker need?

I looped around the park, surprised at the number of people not only also walking but how friendly they were—after a year in this small town I still wasn't used to total strangers saying "Good morning" routinely—and reveled in how nice the park was.

I reveled so much that I lost track of how far I'd gone; when I finally checked my spiffy GPS I realized I was already at 4.8 miles…and still over a mile from home.

Well, that was terrific! I'd gone nearly five miles and only hurt a little bit! My feet ached a bit, and my hips had started to protest around mile four, but I'd done it. Five miles!

But then I had to get home.

Happy enough, I headed down the street, mentally patting myself on the back for hitting five miles without major issues. This whole thing might be a whole lot easier than I ever supposed.

I failed to take into account that I had to keep walking. My brain was already home, but my body was still over a mile from the front door.

At 5.5 miles my hips were screaming at me, and my bladder was poking at me, questioning why I hadn't made use of those neat facilities at the park.

Still more than half a mile to go, and I was in some serious pain, with no one to call to come rescue me from my stupidity, and no place to stop to pee.

I hit the door at 6.25 miles, not wanting to take another step, but having to pretty much run for the bathroom.

Wonderful, I told myself. *We get to do this all over again in the morning.*

Why am I doing this at all?

Max, my psychokitty, cocked his head and looked at me like I was two different kinds of stupid.

Oh yeah. I'm doing it for the boobies.

~

I settled into a routine; I followed the training schedule that was emailed to me every week from the 3 Day website, and four days a week I dragged myself out of bed two to three hours earlier than I normally would, just to get the majority of the miles done before it got too hot.

Once the miles began to pile up, beating the heat became difficult. When August rolled around I was plodding through double-digit weekends, as much as eighteen miles one day and fifteen the next, and I simply didn't have it in me to be up early enough to be done before noon. There was also the matter of being night blind; even if I could have dragged myself out of bed early enough, I wouldn't have been able to see. So I walked in the heat, searching for shade, drinking vast quantities, and most of the time my only issues were blisters and fatigue.

A few times, however, I found myself waged in a mental battle: by mid-afternoon there was little shade to be found as I headed toward home, I couldn't force myself to drink through the nausea, and wondered how I was going to make it home.

Twice I cut my distance in order to be sure I wouldn't collapse on a sidewalk two miles from home; once I cut my mileage because I could feel the sting of a blister beginning to ooze on the bottom of my foot.

But never—and this thrilled me—did I have to stop because of chronic pain. I ached and went through a lot of Ibuprofen and Naprosyn, but it never became so bad that I felt like I couldn't go on.

I wasn't going to say it out loud, lest I jinx myself, but I started to think I had it beat. I might not be cured, but I sure as hell had that monster by the tail and was ready to beat it into a bloody pulp.

~

Aside from the heat, I battled two things during my initial training: blisters and ammonia. The blisters I could understand; even with the magic socks, my feet sweat and the socks got damp. I changed them frequently, but once my mileage began to creep over the 7-8 mile range, I fought blisters on my left foot.

They popped up in the same spots, and only on my left foot, which became a conundrum. I was doing everything right; my shoes fit, I had double-layered wicking socks, I used Body Glide, and I changed my socks every five to six miles. I learned to use Moleskin, double layered it when it felt as if I needed more padding, and still the blisters formed.

Around six weeks before the Walk, I developed the mother of all the blisters I'd ever had, one complete with a baby blister underneath it.

"Soak your feet in tea," Murf told me. "The tannins will help toughen them up."

I wanted to scoff at him, but he was right about the shoes and socks, and he's a runner; he knows a thing or two about foot conditioning.

So I tried it. I bought a kitty litter pan and some cheap generic tea, brewed enough to fill the pan halfway, let it cool, and then soaked my feet every night. I wasn't convinced it would help toughen my feet, but I couldn't deny the fact that it felt good.

After a week or so, I also couldn't deny that the blisters were not only drying out, but the skin on the most sensitive parts of my feet was beginning to thicken a bit. I bolstered it by swabbing my feet with a little bit of Witch Hazel after every walk, and by the time the training miles were winding down, my blisters were under control.

My other battle was less straightforward; after every walk, within minutes of getting home and sitting down, I started smelling ammonia. Initially I thought I smelled cat pee, but it followed me all around the house as I looked for the offender; neither cat could possibly pee that much and neither had ever been prone to spraying; I came to a slow realization that the smell was coming from me.

Wonderful.

I was walking myself into having body odor that smelled a whole lot like I had peed all over myself.

~

"Carb depletion," Murf said. "It happens in some people. You've chewed through your carb reserves, and one of the signs can be that you smell ammonia. It's not a huge concern, unless you start smelling it when you haven't worked out. Eat more carbs along the way."

Easy for him to say.

Somewhere on my laundry list of physical issues is IBS. It's mostly under control, but when I eat and then walk, ugly,

49

ugly things tend to happen. It's a big enough problem that we don't go out to eat if we know we're going to be doing something else afterward; we do whatever else we planned, eat, and then head straight home.

I was already obsessing about how I was going to get through a sixty mile walk with food-and-exercise triggered IBS (Hyperactive Gastrocolic Reflex), but Murf was telling me I needed to address that now, before the 3 Day. The ammonia odor was a symptom telling me I needed more readily available fuel on board.

The most sensible solution was to carry a protein bar with me, but I can't eat soy and every bar we found was loaded with it. Carrying a peanut butter sandwich was doable, but peanut butter gives me hellacious heartburn and I didn't relish the idea of several hours of gnawing burn in my chest. Friends made lists of portable food that addressed both protein and carbohydrate needs, but everything on those lists either contained things I was allergic or sensitive to, or would trigger my gastrocolic reflex.

"You have fast food places along the way," Char said. "Take a chance and experiment. Pick a place to eat, then walk in circles outside until you're sure it won't affect you."

I discovered that I could handle a small McDonald's hamburger without worry, and McD's was located conveniently enough to become my halfway stopping point. It was my longest break during my training walks: stop at McDonald's, eat a burger and drink copiously, go outside and change my socks, check my feet over, change or add Moleskin as needed, and rest a bit. But even when the miles were creeping over twelve at a time, I couldn't fathom eating anything else, even if I was really hungry.

I didn't think there were more than three miles between possible places to stop on the 3 Day, but in real time, that's an hour of walking.

If you're having food-triggered IBS issues, an hour is

problematic.

Hell, fifteen minutes is an issue. I had already been pointed at by a small child as he proclaimed, "Hey, it's that streetwalker lady!" I really didn't want to be known as that streetwalker lady whose intestines had suddenly lacked fortitude right in the middle of Pitt School Road.

~

Eat the burger.

That became somewhat of a mantra; I hated the idea that I was fueling my training walks with a fast food hamburger, but my Irish friend pointed out that it was only 250 calories and had 13 grams of protein. On longer walks I needed the sodium, and I needed food, period.

Apparently, I needed a few more carbs along with that protein.

Across the street from McDonald's is a self-serve frozen yogurt store. I'm lactose intolerant, but I can handle yogurt. That seemed like a handy place to have around, seeing as how I needed more fuel on board. I mapped out my walks so that I stopped a third of the way through at McDonald's, walked a third more, then stopped at Big Spoon for 8-10 ounces of frozen yogurt.

I still smelled ammonia at the end of a long walk, but after some assurances from Murf and a little online research, I decided that since I only smelled it post-workout, and it went away after refueling, I wasn't going to worry about it.

Besides, no one else seemed to be able to smell it on me, and as long as no one else thought I smelled like the litter box, I could live with it.

I was still concerned about what food would do to me on the actual 3 Day walk; I knew I couldn't get away with not eating breakfast, and I wouldn't have my trusty Oatmeal-To-Go square, microwaved for 16 seconds to nice and warm but not too hot, while in camp. I was going to have to rely on the food served, whether it was eggs or cereal or cold lumpy cream of wheat. I was going to have to eat it, and I was going to have to risk whatever might happen.

I contemplated prophylactic Imodium, and wondered if I would wind up with the opposite problem.

I worried more about lunch; after already walking as much as twelve miles, I was sure to be a little nauseous and on the edge of being really tired, and I would have consumed a significant amount of water and electrolyte-enhanced beverages ending in '-ade.' That felt like a recipe for disaster. Overly hungry, over hydrated, overly tired…I had visions of my body exploding in a gross display of Reason #218 Why Thumper Should Not Be Doing This.

My friends' mantra became "You'll be fine."

Granted, they didn't know this, but they said it a lot.

I think they just wanted me to shut up.

* * * *

An aside:

Food along the way during the actual walk was less problematic than every worry I'd had swirling inside my brain suggested to me. There were no McD's burgers being handed out along the way and no giant $1 diet sodas or frozen yogurt, but every two to three miles there was a Pit Stop or Grab-N-Go where I had a choice of chips, fruit, string cheese, water, sports drinks, and Komen Krack.

Yes, Komen Krack.

This is what 3 Day walkers live for: the peanut butter & jelly graham crackers, chilled just enough to keep the peanut butter from being runny. I never would have guessed that I would remotely enjoy PB&J on a cold graham cracker, but let me tell you, those things are so freakishly good that people will hit, kick, scream, pull hair, and cry to get the last one available.

Or maybe that was just me.

I apologize to anyone from whom I may have inadvertently drawn blood. But you have to admit, I have a pretty good round kick, and it's impressive when I can get it head-high.

But yeah…Komen Krack.

I'd been told about the coveted crackers before the first day of the walk but didn't really believe that they were as good as everyone was saying; I worried, too, that one of those 350 calorie wonders would trigger the Really Nasty Things, and contemplated not even trying one. But, we got to the first pit stop and people were going nuts over these things, so I figured I'd at least try it. One bite couldn't hurt, right?

You know what they say about meth? Not even once? They should probably say the same thing about Komen Krack, because one bite and you're doomed. I ate the whole thing and then dreaded the next twenty minutes.

But…I was fine. I noshed my way through day one – not only the PB&J crackers, but through little bags of chips, freakish amounts of candy that people along the way were giving to the walkers, cold crème puffs handed out by employees of a national grocery store chain, some peanut M&Ms I had brought with me, and none of it became an issue.

Nope, IBS related Hyperactive Gastrocolic Reflex was not an issue.

Just the opposite.

But that might be a topic for later…

~

On May 7, 2010, I was invited to join a team of Komen walkers by a blogging cat named Jeter Harris.

On May 10, 2010, Fitness Boy at Fleet Feet in Vacaville, CA fit me for shoes.

On May 11, 2010, I headed out for my very first training walk: three miles that did not kill me. Or maim me. Or even hurt that much. Color me surprised.

On June 8, 2010, just a month after swallowing the fear and registering for the sixty mile walk I was pretty sure I'd never finish, I pounded out eight miles. Granted, my goal for that day had been seven miles, but when I hit that distance I was still a mile from home and just plopping my asterisk down on a curb to wait for someone to come get me didn't seem like a viable option.

Not that I didn't consider it…but it was early enough in the day that I would have waited for at least three hours before Mike would have been awake—he's a night shift vampire—and it could have easily wound up being four hours. Given that the distance back to someplace comfy to sit, like McD's, was almost as far as going home, I opted for home, where I could use my own bathroom, slug back five cans of Diet Cherry Dr Pepper if I so chose, and vegetate in front of the TV.

The distance wasn't lost on me, however. A month earlier if you'd told me I'd walk eight miles in about two and a half hours I'd have snorted derisively and then patted you down for whatever fun stuff you'd been smoking so that I could have some, too.

I also knew that I was going to have to get up the next day and walk another six or seven miles – and it didn't scare me.

One month was all it took; I went from *Oh hell no* to *I can do this*.

Well, I was pretty sure I could do up to ten miles.

Anything more than that scared the snot out of me.

~

Ten days later came the first scheduled ten-mile training walk. I couldn't help but let loose in my head the notion that it had been about ten years since I'd had to use a wheelchair for an entire summer. I couldn't walk ten steps without agony, and there I was ten years later getting ready to head out on a ten-mile walk.

Ten. Ten-ten-ten-ten-ten. More than nine.

Oh Holy Heckola.

I tried to not agonize over the idea. Nine miles was doable; ten seemed impossible. I avoided mentioning my worries to the people who seemed interested in how my training was going, but a few who knew me well knew I had a mental barrier to get over.

"Carb load," Murf said. "Pound down some pasta for dinner the evening before going for the ten. You'll have the energy, I promise."

I was 90% sure he was telling me that in order to push

some of the fear aside, and I was grateful. I wasn't convinced, but I was grateful.

Plus, it was an excuse to have spaghetti, something we rarely had because, face it, pasta is not a diet food, and we were trying to eat well. But for the sake of the ten-mile training walk, we had spaghetti.

Anything for the greater good.

When I headed out on the morning of June 18, I told myself that it would be all right to stop at eight miles if I had to. Eight was technically on the official training schedule, but I'd been pushing it a little, and given what I'd walked the week before, ten miles was on my personal schedule. But, just in case, I mentally prepared myself to deal with falling short and going home at the eight-mile mark.

I will not feel bad, I will not feel bad...

At five miles I stopped at McD's and drank a large Diet Coke as well as some water, and headed back out, sloshing but feeling pretty decent. At 6.5 I still felt all right, and at 7.5 I was still a mile and a half from home, and figured if I was going to do nine I might as well shoot for the ten.

You scheduled ten; you can do ten. Ten! You're gonna walk ten freaking miles!

I may or may not have said that out loud as I walked past a group of mothers and kids playing in the park.

They may or may not have pulled their children closer, away from the crazy lady.

I hit the door at 10.25 miles.

If I hadn't been so sweaty and tired, I would have done the Snoopy Dance right there in the middle of the living room, risking the ridicule and judgment of my cats.

Max the Psychokitty and Buddah Pest, they are harsh critics, indeed.

~

A month later, I was staring at another mental wall. I'd conquered ten miles, but twelve had kicked my ass. The first time I went for twelve, I fell short; I'd taken a break at 5.5 miles, another at 9.5, but by 10.5 I realized I was struggling. My legs hurt, my back was on fire, and the water in my Camelbak was warm and gross tasting. I was half a mile from home and decided to pack it in; twelve was not happening that day, and when I hit the door at 11.2 I decided that was fine and I could live with it.

I tried again the next weekend and made it through with no issues. I didn't think I could have done thirteen, but I managed twelve.

A week later, I did it again, and shaved twenty minutes off my time.

Twelve would be a cakewalk from there on out.

Well.

Two months and roughly a week after this whole training thing started, I dragged my sorry asterisk up at 6:15 in the freaking morning. SIX-FIFTEEN, PEOPLES! It wasn't masochism; the talking heads doing weather on TV all agreed, today would be wicked hot. 100+

So I got up. And I was out the door by 7:15.

The first six miles…not bad at all. It was pleasant out, and I kept finding all kinds of shade to walk in. Some road construction forced me into turning right when I wanted to turn left, but hey, a new route! New things to see and new people to see me walk past and wonder what the heck that old lady was doing wandering around town.

I wound up near Burger King at six miles and went inside for a short break (read: it was .2 miles closer than McD's and I seriously had to pee) and I sat there listening to a group of old people dissect my appearance. They concluded I was probably homeless—I only spent $1 there, after all, and I was kind of grimy looking—and debated whether or not it would be offensive to offer to buy me some breakfast, but before they could come to a conclusion, I got up and went outside to peek at my feet and slap some Moleskin on.

I made a mental note to begin sweating in a less grimy fashion.

The next few miles were not bad at all. It was definitely warming up, but by then I was at the park, where there were lots of trees and some shade to walk through.

At 10.5 miles I was feeling the heat, but hey! Frozen Yogurt RIGHT THERE! How fortunate I just HAPPENED to wind up there right when I was thinking about taking a short break!

But then the ugly started to happen.

At 10.75 miles, the road construction dudes completely blocked the direction I wanted to head in order to get home, and pointed me down a road I did not wish to walk. There was no shade down that street, the sun was beating down, and the temperature was now at Um, Only Morons Are Out Walking Now.

It would also add another mile or two onto my distance.

At eleven miles, I was swearing under my breath, but hey! A street I'd forgotten about, one that cut through some of the worried-about extra distance, was *right in front of me!* So I turned left and was almost happy with the thought that at least I was not going to walk an extra mile.

But my heart rate was up, I was mouth breathing, I was miserable, and I just wanted to get home.

At 11.5 miles, I was looking around to see if there were people nearby; I wanted to be somewhere with other people in case I really was in trouble. I realized the park was just ahead, so instead of going right I went left—same relative distance—because I knew there would be mothers with their spawn at the park, and wouldn't it just make everyone's day if I DROPPED DEAD right in front of the KIDS?

At 11.75 miles I was at the park, muttering to myself, doing a lot of self assessment—HR still higher than usual, but not too high; still mouth breathing but not too hard; I was still sweating and not thirsty—and thinking it *had* to be pushing 100 degrees.

I hit the door right at twelve miles and headed straight for the shower—man, that was gross peeling off sweat soaked clothes—but even after that I was still sweating.

So I checked the thermometer. And then weather.com. Just to see how hard core I am, how much of the hot I can take.

Ninety degrees.

I felt like I was dying and it was only ninety degrees.

I am such a warm weather weenie.

The good news was that it wasn't the distance that got me, it was the fiery furnaces of hell that were blasting down. Because truly, ninety degrees without shade, that's got to be at least an outer circle, right?

Another mental wall went up. Twelve miles had kicked my ass more than once, and I had a thirteen-mile walk to look forward to.

How in the hell?

I chewed on that all week.

Twelve was hard; thirteen was going to kill me.

~

I dreaded it. Twelve miles had kicked my asterisk twice, and I wasn't sure how I'd be able to pull off thirteen. Twelve was my giant wall, the point of No More, and I was about to walk face first into it.

Carb loading wasn't going to fix this. Magic socks and comfy shoes were not the answer. Twelve miles was my limit, and even then I had a hard time with it. Thirteen could not happen.

It just couldn't.

Something had to give.

I couldn't change the distance; I couldn't change the

59

walls I'd walked into. I spent the week musing over what I could change.

The only thing I could change was me.

"It's mental conditioning, not just physical conditioning," Murf's much better half, Char, pointed out.

I'm pretty sure she was kindly telling me that I was mental.

No offense was taken, because I was fairly sure she was right.

On the dreaded morning of I Must Face Thirteen, I got up and decided I was *not* going to walk thirteen miles. I was going to walk three miles, then stop to grab a drink and munch on a granola bar. After that, I would go on a pleasant five-mile walk, then stop for lunch at eight miles total…but at 6.5 I had to sit on a bench in the park to address some foot issues.

I had a particularly bothersome hot spot on my left foot; the Moleskin wasn't helping at all, so I slapped a blister bandage on it, waited a couple of minutes, and got back on my way. I stopped at nine miles for lunch, enjoyed the air conditioning in McDonald's, and then decided to take a 2.5-mile stroll, which I would make sure ended at the frozen yogurt place.

That would put me 1.5 miles from home…for a total of thirteen.

Yep, I molded the day's walk around the idea of eating my way through Dixon.

It worked. By mentally breaking the walk up into smaller chunks, it wasn't this overwhelming idea of walking further than I ever had before. It was just going to get a drink, then going for lunch, then going for dessert, and getting home.

I didn't quite realize it at the time, but I'd put into motion the thing that would get me through the actual 3 Day: I wasn't going to walk sixty miles. I was going to walk five miles…and just do it twelve times.

~

With the majority of the mental walls torn down to a scalable height, I had new issues to deal with.

Blisters.

By the time I was walking thirteen miles, I'd given three different brands of Magic Socks a try. In the first brand I felt like my feet were sweating even more than they ever did in cotton socks, and it felt like my feet were sliding around in my shoes. I gave Thorlos walking socks a try, but felt like they were chewing one spot on my foot, so I switched to Adidas. They were comfortable, but I was still sweating through them. I still had hot spots.

My feet are touchy; I've known that for years. I've never been able to wear a pair of socks more than six or seven times before having to toss them out and buy new; my feet are sensitive enough that I can feel all the little terry-cloth like loops on the inside of socks, which turned out to be the real issue with the Thorlos socks. All I've ever required out of socks is that they feel soft initially, and are cheap.

You can get soft and cheap cotton socks at Walmart.

I knew better than to switch back to cotton, though. If I thought the blisters were bothersome in magic socks, I was pretty sure they'd be raging, blood-filled pustules of agony in cotton.

I needed to toughen my feet up.

This was when Murf coughed up the beverage solution. "Soak your feet in tea."

You have got to be kidding me. Tea? As in the stuff I drink?

Murf was not kidding; the tannic acids in the tea would help to toughen the skin on my feet.

It couldn't hurt; I bought a cheap kitty litter box, some generic tea, brewed up a giant pan full, and once it had cooled I soaked my tired feet in it. The cats were extremely interested in this, and their attention to where my feet were added a new wonder: how badly would it smell if either of them decided to pee in my tea box?

I kept it covered with plastic, just in case, and brewed a new batch every few days.

Even if it didn't help toughen my feet, it felt good and smelled wonderful.

The next weekend I tackled fourteen miles on Friday and then ten on Saturday. The next week I walked fifteen on Friday and eleven on Saturday, and was feeling pretty confident about how the rest of my training would go. I wasn't looking forward to the next bump in miles, which would have me walking seventeen miles one day and thirteen the next, but I also wasn't afraid of it.

Oddly, I was looking forward to it.

The beginning of August had me feeling tired but confident, and after my fifteen and eleven mile weekend I began planning out the next week: what to do for cross-training, where I would walk on my shorter-mile days. Maybe go to San Francisco, walk the hills there. Maybe find someplace in Sacramento to walk, something different.

I was making all kinds of plans.

But then my father died, and I really didn't care if I walked another training mile or not.

* * * *

My father's death was not unexpected; he'd been steadily declining for a long time and my sisters kept me apprised of his condition. Still, it was a sucker punch to the gut and walking was the last thing on my mind. The only thing I had in front of me was getting on a plane and going to Texas for his funeral.

The bigger picture didn't keep me from noticing while walking through airports that I was having some significant blister issues. They were ugly and didn't feel any better than they looked; I sucked it up and tried to not think about the pain on the bottom of my foot as we made our way through airports, to the hotel, and through his funeral. I acknowledged it on the way home, but only because by then everything was annoying me.

The day after coming home, the blisters opened, drained, and began to dry out.

I decided my dad had a hand in that, and tried to put my head back into training for the 3 Day.

The upcoming weekend called for seventeen miles one day and thirteen the next; if the blisters healed over I was fairly sure I could do the seventeen-mile walk, but was a little less confident about following it up the following day with thirteen. It was time to check out new Magic Socks; before leaving for Texas I'd done a bit of researching online and found several recommendations for Wrightsocks double layered running socks, and they seemed to make sense for me. Mike called around to local shoe stores and found one in Sacramento, about thirty miles away, so we headed up there and bought three pairs to try.

Two days after coming home, I headed out on a five-mile walk with my hopefully spiffy new Magic Socks; I didn't want to count that distance as being much of anything, just as getting back into the swing of things. And I didn't want to base the success of the socks on it, because the rather large blister on the bottom of my left foot had popped, revealing a blister underneath it – some healing had to happen before I could declare the socks a success or a failure.

I kept walking, kept an eye on the blisters, and looked ahead to the weekend. Blisters or not, seventeen miles had to happen.

~

During a Komen 3 Day, you're not allowed to use ear buds or headphones, or anything else (like cell phones) that might block your ability to hear the things going on around you. It's a safety issue and I understood that from the beginning; they want you to be able to hear that out-of-control SUV that's about to plow you off the side of the road.

Since most of my training was done alone, I often listened to music, using only one ear bud in order to have the other ear free to hear screeching brakes and screams of *Oh My Gawd, Move!* coming from all around me. With an entire day of walking ahead of me (and I was certain that seventeen miles would take me most of the day) I wanted something different and distracting, so I downloaded an audiobook.

Peoples, I wish I'd done that from the beginning. It was easy to lose myself in the book; I didn't forget I was plodding along at three miles an hour, but it was definitely more enjoyable.

Seventeen miles made my feet sore, but I didn't pop up a new blister, and I ended it looking forward to the next day because I had a really good book to finish.

It's worth noting that if you're listening to something really funny, you're going to get a lot of odd looks from people you pass.

My feet held up just fine the next day; they were sore

but that was it. No new blisters bubbled up and I noticed no major hot spots. But the rest of me?

Engrossing books aside, I hurt on that walk.

A lot.

I'd woken up at 4 a.m. with a ropy pain behind one knee, and by the time I got up I was seriously debating whether to walk or not.

I loaded up on Naprosyn and walked. And at five miles I was sucking down Motrin.

At seven miles I sat down on the first bench I could find for a few minutes, mentally calculating the distance from there to home.

I sat down again at eight miles, because my hips were joining in on the fun.

Again at nine, thanks to my back.

I took a longer break at ten.

Sat down at 11.5…and then shuffled the rest of the way home. I walked slowly all day; it took me about forty minutes longer than it should have, and I spent a good part of the day wondering how the hell I'd be able to do two twenty-mile days, much less three.

Nearly every step I took that day sucked hard and was lead-weighted with doubt.

It's mental conditioning, not just physical conditioning.

I pondered that, and mentioned to Murf that his wife was in my head. He agreed with her: most of what I had to push through was all the clatter spinning through my brain. Physically, if I'd survived thirty miles in two days I could do sixty miles in three. After all, it was just three miles further on one day and seven the next; the third day I'd be walking fueled by adrenaline and I'd be surrounded by people who would help boost me up along the way. I needed to get over this mental hump.

I needed, he said, to understand why I was doing it. And then he asked me point blank: *why are you doing this?*

I thought about it.
I pondered it.
Then I blogged about it.

~

Simple enough question. "Why are you doing this?"

Look, I've kind of expected that question all along and have had a pat answer: nothing I've gone through—none of the chronic pain (I'm not proud, I'll list it: Fibromyalgia, Chronic Myofascial Pain, and arthritis in my lower spine and in both hips), the months in the wheelchair, the brain tumor, the marathon peeing and drinking and wondering when the hell my meds will kick in, or worse when they'll wear off—has been half as hard as someone else hearing they have breast cancer, and then what they go through in treatment. The chemo. The radiation.

It sounds like a great answer, right? Doing this long walk because even when you add it onto everything else, it still seems insignificant.

But before I could type out my pat answer, I was hit with, "And don't give me any of the typical bullshit. I don't really need to know why you're doing it. YOU need to know why you're doing it."

Well...fine. Color me stumped and momentarily speechless.

"Don't tell me either that you're doing it because The Grate Jeter Harris Hizself's mom asked you to. Why are YOU doing it?"

The person posing the question? He doesn't really expect an answer. He's the kind of person that asks random crap just to make other people ponder themselves. I imagine he asks himself random crap like this all the time, just for the exercise of self-introspection. I imagine he asks his wife things all the time to just get her to stop in time and in place for a moment, to simply consider.

I had plenty of time over the weekend to ponder the why of it all. I distracted myself from the sheer number of steps required to complete 17 and then 13 miles with a really good audiobook, but that didn't keep my brain from working in the background while I was listening to Joshilyn Jackson read her own work. The last two miles of Saturday's 17 hurt like hell, and I pondered it over and over.

What the hell am I doing to myself?

When I got up Sunday morning and had knee pain that rated an 8 on a 1-10 scale, I briefly considered not walking at all. Why go through the pain? After all, this is the training portion; this isn't the "real walk."

Except that it is.

I got up and walked, not because I'm a masochist, and not because I'm some wonderful person who said she'd do it, so she's doing it. I got up and walked because all the steps leading up to The Walk count. They're part of the process. They're part of the bigger picture. They're just as real as It is.

I'm not kidding anyone; this training is kicking my ass, and it fucking hurts. That pain you feel the first day after starting a new exercise routine? I start from there. My best days start from some version of that. I knew that when I accepted the invitation to sign up for this walk, and I decided to do it in spite of it.

And the truth is that I didn't say I'd do it because getting a diagnoses of cancer is harder than anything I've gone through; I didn't do it because chemo and radiation and mastectomy are more difficult. When it comes down to it, I wanted to do this because what I've gone through has been hard. It's been gut wrenchingly hard, and it's been *fuckit-am-I-going-to-die?* hard.

Hearing a bad diagnosis? I've been there. I remember what it felt like to be told I had a tumor clinging to the underside of my brain, and that it was big. I remember the dread of being told that because it was big, and because they just couldn't tell from the MRI exactly what type of tumor it was—something harmless or something insidious—that it had to come out; I know now how fear drips from your fingertips in electric slivers. I will never forget the feeling of checking into the hospital and just *not knowing.* How badly will this hurt? How long will it take? Will I wake up and hear "Sorry, but it sucks to be you"? Will I wake up at all? I still feel the resignation of knowing that I wasn't getting out of it, that someone was going to reach into my head and cut something out, and if I bolted it just meant more uncertainty.

Will I live, or will I die?

I've done hard.

I don't want other people to do hard.

I don't want some 20-something young woman who hasn't even started her life to have to face anything that hard. Or some 20-something young man. Or 30 or 40-something. 90-something.

This wouldn't even have to be a walk for breast cancer. My mother had lymphoma; I could easily do a walk for the Leukemia and Lymphoma Society, and I may at some point. Hell, I probably will. My father had kidney cancer. I could easily walk for symptom awareness, how to save your own life.

It's all hard. It's all fucking hard.

But this? I can *do* this. If any or every step I take means there's a small chance that someday someone else won't have to sit there and hear about some wayward thing growing in their body, that's some of the why of it all.

The possibilities.

The *hope*.

That doesn't make me some Pollyanna tightass halo-glowing wonderdork; I'm not doing anything thousands upon thousands of other people aren't doing and haven't already done this year. Hell, if I hadn't been asked to join a team, it never would have crossed my mind. And when I was asked, it scared the hell out of me.

Because I knew it would be hard.

I will probably find myself weighed down with more doubts over the next month; the next long walk weekend is 18 miles one day and (I think) 15 the next. It's going to hurt, and I'm going to complain about it. Not whine, but complain, because it's going to hurt, and it's going to be hard.

The thing is, hard isn't fatal.

Why am I doing it? I think the answer is because I need to know that I *can*. That everything that's been hard hasn't been in vain. So that I can say I damn well did it.

It's a selfish motivation.

:::shrugs:::

I can live with that.

~

The walk I'd signed up for was scheduled for the first weekend in October; toward the end of August, during the week of my birthday, Mike took time off and we headed for San Francisco. We wanted to wander around, do touristy things, but there were other motivations.

Namely, hills.

The 3 Day was in San Francisco, so it made sense to get away from the flatness of Dixon roads and sidewalks and start some decent hill training – and where better than in San Francisco itself?

San Francisco has hills. Lots and lots of hills. It's almost like some sadist sat down in city planning a couple hundred years ago, rubbed his hands together while cackling, and declared this would be the most painful city *ever* to walk around in. People will come to visit, and the things they'll take away with them are shin splints and an overwhelming sense of badassness for having survived them all.

What San Francisco lacks in flatness, it makes up for in scenery. In a relatively small geographical area you can go from the crowds and heavy traffic of a loud, bustling downtown to the serenity and beauty of waves lapping onto the beach in less than ten miles. You can hike through woods, walk along the Golden Gate Bridge, visit incredibly lush parks, and even wander around the downtrodden and somewhat scary neighborhood of the Tenderloin.

San Francisco has it all, and in a couple of days you can see it all. It's amazing, and a damn near perfect place for someone to go to train to walk hills. Any effort is made easier by the sights, something that ancient city planner probably knew.

On my 49th birthday we drove to the city to see the Golden Gate Bridge and walked halfway across; it was cold and windy, the fog rolling overhead and hiding the tips of the bridge's supports. I stood there shivering on the bridge, watching a freighter make its way into the Bay, and decided that Mark Twain was right. The coldest winter one might spend is a summer day in San Francisco.

We hopped back into the car and fought our way through traffic to downtown, found spendy parking, and then wandered around Union Square. We shopped without buying anything, dodged the panhandlers and people handing out religious tracts. It was a blast, but we ran out of time to see as much as we would have liked, and decided to come back to do some real walking in a few days.

The week of my birthday, we did a lot of walking. There were no formal training walks; we went to Six Flags and spent the day wandering around there, not getting on rides, just walking between Things to See. We went to a flea market in Sacramento and spent the day walking around that. Three days after the first trip to San Francisco we went back.

This time we took the Bay Area Rapid Transit train (BART) to avoid the choke of city traffic; it afforded us the chance to just walk around without having to find a place to park (and to avoid paying out the nose for parking) and to not worry about the likely two hours it would take getting out of downtown and onto the Bay Bridge during rush hour.

We decided to spend part of the day just walking—I needed to get a good idea how killer those hills were going to be—and then part of the day being tourists. We wandered up Powell Street ("up" being the key word there) and then through Chinatown, gradually making our way towards the Bay and Ghiradelli Square. From there we wandered along the Wharf, to Pier 39 (giant tourist magnet that can magically empty out your wallet) and then did the ultimate in touristy things: got on a cable car and took it the three miles back to where we started.

Other than a couple of eighteen and fifteen mile training

walks, I didn't embark on any seriously long walks after that. I concentrated on those hills, and we went back to San Francisco at least once a week after that; up a hill for a few blocks, walk laterally for a block or two, up another hill. We walked through Chinatown and all the shops, walked around Union Square and down to Market Street and back up again; it was walking without feeling like training, and it was wonderful.

It was the last training puzzle piece to fall into place. I was no longer worried about the actual 3 Day. I would either walk sixty miles, or I wouldn't. I would have to take a sweep van at some point, or I wouldn't. My feet would hold up, or they wouldn't.

I'd trained, I'd raised the funds, and I was as ready as I could be, so there was no point in worrying about walking.

No, I had a whole other host of things I was beginning to chew on.

Food…I have food allergies. I really didn't want to unwittingly ingest a stealth mushroom and then suffer the after effects. I don't go into anaphylaxis; I just get sick. Very, very sick, with wonderful eruptions from every available bodily orifice. Mango or kiwi, those might kill me. A banana? My tent mate better pray I didn't eat one, though it might solve a heat issue.

I could pretty much guarantee that one banana and we'd be warm all night.

I worried about my medications and how well they would work. Normally if the meds for my diabetes insipidus wear off early I just sit at home and drink and pee; if it wore off during the walk…? I wasn't sure I would be able to get enough to drink or if I would be able to make it from one pit stop to the next without peeing myself.

Oh, walking was no longer the issue.

Bodily fluids? That was another matter.

~

With only a month to go until the first day of the 3 Day, I found my excitement ratcheting up. I was ready for it, mentally and physically, determined to not let worries about food get in my way, and was willing to swallow whole my own natural shyness.

I'd only met one person on my team, so this fell into the realm of Big Freaking Deal for me; what saved my sanity was knowing there were several people on the team, so I was probably going to be able to be quiet without anyone taking offense, and besides…these were, for the most part, cat bloggers and people who liked cat bloggers.

I might be socially backwards, but I would survive.

I kept walking, sometimes around the outlet mall in Vacaville for variety, sometimes in San Francisco, a lot of the time near home, where I was becoming a fixture around town. At McDonald's the cashier noticed if I was missing my white baseball cap, people in the park sometimes inquired about the day's mileage, and one small boy squealed to his mother, "It's that streetwalker lady!"

I learned the layout of our small town. By the time my training was winding down, I could tell you how far it was from point A to point B from almost any starting point. When asked for directions—and that was frequent—I could answer with a precision that left some people amused. Surely she can't be serious when she says to go eight tenths of a mile down the street, turn left, drive one and one quarter miles, turn right, and then in one eighth of a mile, there's the Super Walmart.

It's a small town; one lap equals five miles. That's it.

More importantly, I knew my own landscape. I knew what I could take. I knew how I'd feel if I went down Pitt School Road at 10 am, and how different I would feel at 3 pm. I knew my tolerances, I knew my preferences, and most of all, I knew I could, and would, do it.

ROCK THE WALK

I live roughly fifty miles from San Francisco and theoretically could have gotten up at Way Too Early o'clock on the first day of the 3 Day and left my car at the Cow Palace, where the opening ceremony was being held, but fifty miles between here and the Bay Bridge could take anywhere from two to three hours, and besides, my teammates—most of whom I had never met—were staying at the host hotel and we'd planned a pre-walk team dinner.

It was easier to stay at the host hotel; I could meet my friends for dinner and not have a two to three hour ride home, only to have to repeat it in the morning.

Mike took the weekend off to go with me; he wanted to meet the women I was walking with, and he wanted to be there for the opening ceremony and to cheer us as we got underway. I wondered how he'd feel being surrounded by hundreds of women in the hotel, but one of the first walkers we saw as we checked in was a tall, burly guy.

Wearing a hot pink bra.

Over his black t-shirt.

The hotel lobby was swarming with women in pink: pink tutus, pink t-shirts, pink deely-boppers on their heads, pink everything, but it was men that stood out.

The other thing that stood out: these are not shy people. It didn't matter that I'd never seen any of them before, I was there in my pink Komen shirt and obviously walking or crewing, therefore I was now A Friend.

A year later, in Atlanta, I would come to appreciate that in a way I never realized I would, but for the time being it was simply amusing.

~

Can I do it?

That's not an absurd question; I've heard some absurd answers to it, answers that range from the guilt inducing *There are people out there dying from breast cancer and you wonder whether or not you can walk?* to the borderline snobbish *Maybe not; this is a very difficult thing to do and not everyone is cut out for it.*

The question itself is worth asking of oneself.

My take on it after having done the training for three walks now? Sure, you can do it. With few exceptions, your weight, physical condition, height, hair color, income, and addiction to dark chocolate and purple fuzzy things are not impediments to walking sixty miles in three days. I admit, during my first walk I was surprised at the variety of people huffing and puffing right along with me; there were the thin, fit, perky women bobbing along effortlessly, but there were just as many people like me: overweight, not in the best shape, with physical conditions that could be used as valid reasons for not even thinking about this walk. There were women with canes, with pronounced limps; there were women obese enough that I did honestly question the wisdom of them attempting this.

I don't know if any of them made use of the sweep vans, but it doesn't matter whether they did or not; they were there, and they undoubtedly trained for it.

On my second walk there was a younger woman in a

wheelchair, accompanied by her mother and father, who pushed her up the hills and kept her from rolling out of control down the hills.

On my third walk, there was more than one wheelchair participant, at least one woman walking with a broken foot, and a couple of *very* pregnant women.

The answer to the question of "Can I do it?" is yes.

The next question should be "Should I do it?"

The answer to that is a big fat "Maybe…"

While pretty much everyone is capable of tackling the training required to get through walking twenty miles a day for three days straight, not everyone has the time. In the initial stages you only need a few hours a week to dedicate to it, but when you're coming into those last couple of months before the walk, you very nearly need entire days; once you're walking twelve miles a day, and then hitting the weeks where you're walking fifteen miles one day and twelve the next—leading up to eighteen and fifteen—you need time.

If you have kids and no one to watch them, your training will suffer.

If you have a job that precludes that kind of time, your training will suffer.

Should you feel bad about that?

No. Absolutely not.

You may still be able to walk; it just depends on how you feel about the training that you are able to do, and whether or not you have issues with taking a sweep van during the 3 Day. There are plenty of people who only train a couple of days a week, doing only one long walk in combination with shorter mileage days and cardio training. I've met a couple of people who barely train; they're in excellent physical condition and just go for it. Sometimes they can do all twenty miles each day, other times they can't, and they're fine with that.

If you can't walk, there are other ways you can get involved. Charity walks like the Komen 3 Day need warm bodies as support; if you can't walk, you can volunteer as part of the crew. In fact, if you have certain specialties—EMT, RN, chiropractor, physician—you may be far more valuable to the cause if you volunteer your services for the event.

If you can't walk or crew, you can show up and cheer for the walkers. I can't even begin to describe how wonderful it is to turn a corner and suddenly have a dozen people literally cheering because you're out there walking. The people who show up and support the walkers are every bit as important as the crew; when you're on mile seventeen and you're just about out of gas, having people there who are hooting and hollering, handing out candy and high fives, can add a little fuel to the tank.

But let's go on the premise that you intend to walk; you have the time, you can raise the minimum funds, and you want to be part of the effort that eventually finds a cure, and make a huge difference along the way.

You want to know what it's going to be like, right?

It's going to be amazing.

The Host Hotel

For every walk, there is a host hotel; there may be more than one hotel with special rates arranged for by the 3 Day, but typically there's one main hotel, from which you'll be able to catch a bus to the opening ceremony on Friday morning; that's the hotel you want to stay at. Unless you live within an easy drive to the site of opening at your walk, and have someone who can drop you off, I highly recommend staying at the host hotel the night before the walk begins. That means paying close attention to the 3 Day website and being ready to make reservations as soon as they announce the hotel for your city; rooms go quickly and if you hesitate, you run the risk of not getting a room there. If you don't get into one of the rooms reserved for the 3 Day, you don't get a shuttle pass to opening, and then you wind up having to take a taxi, figure out the bus lines, or beg a ride from someone.

I've done—as of this writing—three 3 Day events; two in San Francisco and one in Atlanta. The hotels for both were *nice*. The prices weren't half bad, either; the event coordinators tend to get some very good rates on the rooms, and if you share with other walkers you can really cut the price down. Both hotels were in the $200 range for a room (or suite) with two queen beds, when the normal rate would have run closer to $400. Four walkers to a room, $50.

If you're part of a team, room sharing is easy; if you're not, it's still doable. Get online and scope out the message boards, look for out-of-towner info for the city in which you're walking. People often post to find others who want to share rooms, or you can ask if there's anyone out there who wants to share. I wouldn't worry too much about getting ripped off; after all, you're going to know where each other will be for the next three days.

Some host hotels offer a special event dinner the night

before the walk; in San Francisco the hotel had a pasta meal for around $15. The hotel for Atlanta 2011 had no organized dinner, but they did have an upscale Italian restaurant and two informal dining options. I would advise getting online and checking out the dining options within easy walking distance to the hotel before leaving home; the food in Atlanta was tasty, but pricey, and if not for the people I was meeting, I would have chosen something close by or even delivery if it was available.

Eat dinner early, and get back to your room at a reasonable time; you're going to be getting up at O'Dark:thirty on Friday morning.

Participating in San Francisco spoiled me a bit; the host hotel there offered—at no additional cost—a continental type breakfast, and they have food ready and waiting by 3:30 a.m., early enough for crew members to grab breakfast before they leave at 4 a.m. We were surprised in Atlanta; there was a breakfast buffet, but at $13 per person it wasn't worth it. There was also a coffee shop in the hotel that several walkers made use of, but at 5:30 in the morning, not everyone was thinking clearly, and a bunch of us spent a little too much for gooey buffet style cheesy scrambled eggs and fruit.

Yep, it's an early start to the day. You'll be getting up around 4-4:30 in the morning to get dressed, repack your bag, and grab some food before getting on the shuttle bus that will take you to opening, which begins between 7-7:30 in the morning. And trust me, you want to be there for opening ceremonies.

OPENING CEREMONY

Chances are you'll get on the shuttle at the hotel between 5:30-6:45 in the morning; if you're worried that you'll be half in the bag from lack of sleep, don't gnaw on that nugget of concern too much. Once you hit the hotel lobby, the atmosphere will be swollen with excitement, and by the time you hand your under-35-pound bag off to be shoved into bus cargo, ride the bus to the opening ceremony site, recover and then take your under-35-pound bag to the energetic, smiling, very helpful crew members who will haul your belongings onto one of several trucks, and then wander to where the actual ceremony will be, you're going to be wide awake and ready to get going.

No matter how prepared you are, you want to be there a little early; if you've already checked in online, have your water bottles filled, feet prepped, and have the things you think you'll need throughout the day right where you can easily get to them in your waist pack or backpack, you might think there will be nothing to do until it all begins. Plus, you want to get going. This is what all those training miles have been leading up to. Let's just skip the whole thing and get going already!

If you didn't check in online or you didn't print out your credentials—that's an important little piece of paper—head for the check-in tent. You need to get that done before you do anything else. You'll be carrying the credentials with you on the entire walk on a lanyard; you need to show those to be scanned onto the route and then back into camp, and having them hanging around your neck is quick I.D. if something happens along the way. You'll also get your tent assignment, which will be printed on your credentials.

Once you do that, there are things to do, things you'll

want to be a part of. There is always a 3 Day store at the opening ceremony site, so you can buy a t-shirt or beads, event pins or a hat – just remember that unless you have a non-walker to whom you can give your purchases for safekeeping you'll be carrying what you've bought all day. The 3 Day store will also be open at camp, but some people prefer to buy things before the event begins, because some items sell out quickly and they don't want to risk it. But you will have an opportunity to shop at camp.

One of the first things I look for is the table with the memorial flag laid over it; this is the flag upon which you can write the names of those you've lost to breast cancer. There might not be a sign directing walkers to it, but you'll be able to tell what it is at a glance. In the past it's been comprised of inch-wide strips of cloth, but in 2011 it was one long white single cloth. If you see people hunched over a table while they write, you've probably spotted the memorial flag. Take a minute and add any names of the people you miss.

There's also a wall upon which you can place stickers with the reasons you're walking; it can be those very same names you wrote upon the memorial flag, or it can be for someone who is alive and fighting. It can be uniquely personal—to just do it, to stare down fear, to set an example for your kids—or you can write down a favorite saying. Quote lyrics. Draw a happy face. Anything that has meaning for you.

The wait before the start of the opening ceremony is a good time for team and individual pictures, too; there will be a wall where you and your teammates can take a Day 1, 0-Mile photo; sometimes there are crew members who will take your camera and snap pictures for you, but if there's no crew, the person in line behind you will happily do it. You'll probably be asked to take five pictures with five different cameras, and trust me, you won't mind at all.

Twenty minutes or so before the ceremony begins (and

you still might be thinking you just want to skip everything and get going to get those first miles behind you) the corral near the stage where the walkers congregate for the opening ceremony is opened. You won't just be standing around shuffling from one foot to the other while you wait; music is blaring, and the beach balls come out.

Yep, beach balls.

Giant pink and white beach balls.

This is truly a time when your head will be tested for its beach-ball-magnetic properties. My skull happens to be seriously BBM; even if I'm paying attention to where all the balls are—and there are usually six or seven of them bouncing around—I get bonked on the head half a dozen times.

At least, I'm pretty sure it was my magnetic personality that pulled the balls toward me. Surely people were not deliberately spiking them my way.

Don't be shy; if one of those balls heads in your direction, go for it. Slap it back into the air and keep it going. It's a fun way to get things started and once everyone has been bouncing the balls around for ten minutes or so, out comes Stretching Boy (or Stretching Girl) to the stage. The balls get put away and the crowd gets down to business; you're about to embark on a long day of walking and ideally you need to stretch. Who knew the fun with the beach balls was to help you get warmed up?

The operative word in regard to stretching here is "ideally." When you have 1500-4000 people packed into a relatively small space, getting a really good stretch is a bit difficult. It's doable, but some of the stretches are a little difficult to manage when you only have a few inches of space in which to maneuver.

Try anyway.

You want to be good and warmed up, stretched out, and ready, because you're about to be soaked in emotion.

More accurately, you're about to be flagged with a cacophony of sadness, admiration, awe, sympathy, empathy, and determination. Once Stretching Boy is done with you, the ceremony begins, and it begins with the flags.

The flags are reminders of everything we're walking for, carried by fellow walkers and crew members, a subtle yet in-your-face message. We're walking to raise money in the fight against breast cancer, but there's so much more. The flags that will be carried around the corral of eager walkers speak of the things for which we're undertaking this adventure: anniversaries, graduations, weddings, dreams, and more. They remind us of the people for whom we walk: My Grandmother, My Mother, My Sister, My Aunt, My Father.

Yes, there's a My Father flag. People tend to forget that men get breast cancer, too; we lose somewhere between 400-500 men to the disease every year.

We might be awash in pink, but we walk for men, too.

After the flag bearers have come across the stage and formed a circle around the walkers, you're going to get some very vivid, very human reminders of what's really at stake and the potential that every step of the walk brings: the survivors. In what will likely be one of the most solemn and stark moments of the entire event, breast cancer survivors bearing their flags will cross the stage and enter a raised island in the middle of the crowd. They will raise the memorial flag as we all take a few moments to remember the names we wrote on that flag.

You're there for a purpose.

You're not just there to raise money. You're not just there to walk until your feet feel like they're going to fall off. You're not just there because you had a free weekend and it's something fun to do.

You're there because you don't want to see another person die from this disease.

You will choke back a few tears—or let them freely fall—and then you'll suck in a deep breath. All those training miles, all the effort you put into this, the headaches of getting the rest of your life accomplished while you trained, it has an even deeper meaning now.

You'll carry that sense of purpose with you, through the rest of the opening ceremony, though the incredibly moving speech that will set your nerves on fire and whip you into truly being ready to go, and that sense of purpose will explode into excitement the moment you hear, "The Susan G. Komen 3 Day begins right NOW!"

DAY 1

If you're closest to the stage during the opening ceremony, you'll be among the first walkers let out of the corral and onto the route. If you're not, prepare to meet other walkers up close and personal. The electric excitement of finally starting has people pushing to move forward and to stay with their friends and teammates. I've never heard of anyone being trampled, so it's probably not something one should put on their list of things to worry about; it's just something you might want to be aware of. If getting out onto the route early is important to you, try to be near the stage. If you don't care, be toward the back of the crowd.

No matter where you are, as you make your way toward the beginning of day one's route, you're going to be cheered loudly, offered a few hundred high fives, and it's going to hit you: this is a Big Freaking Deal! And that's before you're even officially scanned onto the route (remember the credentials? This is when you need them.)

~

You're off. You're walking. You're bouncing along with a stream of people ahead of you (unless you're the lead walker, in which case, I hate you but not really) and a stream of people behind you (unless you're the last walker, in which case I love you and I really mean that) and even though it's still WayTooEarly in the morning, this is awesome. Not just "Whoa, dude!" awesome, but the literal definition of the word.

Hundreds, even thousands, of men and women walking en masse, for the same cause, and you can't imagine it being any better.

Then someone driving by honks.

Another car honks.

The next car, the driver not only honks but is also waving like crazy at you all. People are opening their windows and yelling *You go girl!* Then you make note of the car of college-age boys hanging out their car windows, wearing funky hats, and they're shouting for you—not at you—and honking like madmen. The car is covered in support graffiti: *We Love Boobies! Free Mammograms Here! I Honk for Hooters!* Those kids ride the route all day, their support never waning.

Before you're five miles out, you're probably going to see the first of the community support. There will be drivers honking at you all day long, and I like to think those are people who get it. Who appreciate what you're doing.

And, granted, a few of them probably just like honking at a bunch of women, but still…for the first few hours, you're going to get a kick out of it. Smile and wave. You'll make their day, too.

Along the route there are designated cheering stations, places where you can have friends and family meet you, where they can bring signs and pom poms, where they can scream and shout, jump up and down, do backflips – whatever they want to do to cheer the walkers on. But even between those official cheering stations you're going to come across locals who know the route and who camp out all day long to support you.

These lovely people are one of the reasons you will lose absolutely no weight while walking for three days. They will give you candy, lots and lots of candy, and sometimes cookies, fruit, or bottled water. Right about the time you've resolved to take no more candy, there will be little kids standing on the sidewalk holding out tootsie rolls in their little fists, and you just can't bear to tell them you don't need anything at the moment.

Some people are especially organized in their cheering efforts. When I walked in Atlanta in 2011, there were groups that showed up every day in multiple locations, offering hot coffee and freshly baked bread to the walkers. One family was there every afternoon, handing out ice-cold soft drinks (and for a Diet Coke addict such as myself that was extraordinarily sweet. I told the little old boy who gave me a Diet Coke that I loved him…I think I freaked him out a little.)

In some cities, too, you'll find that businesses—some national chain stores, some small and local—have people out there handing out goodies. In San Francisco a national grocery store chain hands out cold crème puffs and popsicles. On my first walk there was a national big box store handing out small smoothies. And one of the more creative and very much appreciated things given out by a small local store: baby wipes. Late in the afternoon, when we were all sweaty and tired and kind of stinky, we passed by a couple sitting outside their store; each held out a pop-up baby wipe dispenser for walkers to take as they needed.

Trust me, my pits needed.

It's a sixty mile buffet line. No, you will not lose weight.

~

Roughly every three miles, there will be a pit stop. At these you'll have access to the world's cleanest port-a-potties, water and sports drinks, chips, fruit, string cheese, candy, and peanut butter and jelly graham crackers – Komen Krack. There will also be a medical tent where you can sit to check blisters and care for them if needed, and there will be medical personnel on hand if you need to be seen.

Don't be stoic; if your muscles hurt abnormally, you feel shin splints coming on, or especially if you feel nauseous and achy—if there's any chance you might be dehydrated and/ or your electrolytes are off—stop at the medical tent. Don't worry that they'll pull you off the walk; unless your blisters look serious or you're in real trouble from dehydration, they won't. But if they do, it's because you need to stop. Listen to them, do what they say. They're not there to make your walk suck, they're there to make your walk safe.

Pit stops are a good place to take a few minutes to stretch, too. Granted, you can stretch a bit at every stoplight that holds you up along the way, but if you're like me you don't necessarily make the best use of that time, so take it at the pit stops.

Your muscles will thank you in the morning.

Along with the pit stops, there are also a few Grab-N-Go stations along the walk. Here you can use a port-a-potty and grab water and sports drinks, and get on your way quickly. But if you feel like you need to rest for a few minutes, then take the time. The people who get ahead of you aren't going to use all the miles; they'll leave you plenty.

Your longest stop will probably be at lunch (which can be anywhere from mile nine to mile fourteen), and if you walked enough training miles in preparation for this, by the time you hit the lunch stop, you'll still be feeling fine. Blisters happen, leg cramps happen, but in general, as long as you've trained and you've kept hydrated along the way, the only thing you'll be at lunch is hungry and a little tired. You'll also have found your groove and know what to expect for the rest of the day.

Walk, drink, eat, drink, pee, eat, drink, pee. What, candy for ME? Walk-walk-walk-eat-drink-pee-drink-pee.

Pretty much like that.

By mile sixteen on Day One the thought that this needs to end soon might begin to leak out of your subconscious and into your brain. You also might feel a bit concerned because you've walked this far several times before and not felt nearly as tired or ready to stop, but it's normal. You've done sixteen to seventeen miles and felt fine, but you hadn't been riding on a wave of excitement for the first ten to twelve of those miles before. You'd probably also gotten a full night's sleep and hadn't been stuffing yourself with candy all day.

Drink, stretch, and keep going. It's going to be fine and you're not that far from the end of the day's walking.

Your first day you will probably do between twenty and twenty-two miles, and when you get scanned into camp your first thought might be *oh holy carp I need a shower!* But truly, that's not what you want to do.

Besides, you have a few other things you need to do first.

Yep, you've walked over twenty miles, and you still have things to do.

~

Once you get to camp on day one, you need to retrieve your bag, grab a tent, find your assigned tent spot, and then set your tent up. If you know that the person you're tenting with is already in camp, you might be able to skip the picking up of the tent and go straight to your camp spot, but if you've been assigned to tent with a stranger, you might want to go see if they've already been there and set it up for you.

Let's assume they have not.

First off, don't worry about how difficult it is to put the tent up; I've talked to a few people who seriously worried about that for weeks before the walk. "I can barely put Legos together, how can I put a tent together and get it to stay up?" It's a legitimate concern if you've never camped before, but there are clear directions packed in with the tent, and it will take fewer than five minutes to erect. As soon as you have it up, put something in it, because they are very lightweight and will float off in a slight breeze. After walking all day, you really don't want to be the person running after a tumbleweed tent.

Something worth noting: you want a tarp under your sleeping area to keep your mattress, sleeping bag and anything else in the tent dry in case of rain. I've seen a lot of people put the tarp under the tent, but it's probably better to put the tarp inside, on the tent floor. Yes, *inside* the tent.

If it rains, water will drip down the sides of the tent, and if you've placed the tarp under it, water will pool on its edges and when that happens, it seeps under the tent – not under the tarp, but between it and the tent. End result: the water seeps through and your stuff gets wet.

If you place the tarp on the floor inside the tent, when that water drips and then works its way under the tent, you still have a barrier between it and your things. You don't need a heavy duty, pricey tarp; shower curtains from the dollar store work well. A rolled plastic painting dropcloth, which you can get for about a dollar at Walmart, is effective and you won't even worry about getting it rolled back up to take home (I'm not sure if it's done in every city, but I've noted on two walks that there have been donation piles near gear turn-in, and you can leave your tarp there.)

The tents are on the small side: 6.5 x 6.5 and if you have two twin sized air mattresses inside, there's really no room for anything else. That includes your bag. Chances are you'll wind up storing your bag outside the tent, and for that I highly recommend using clear contractor-grade trash bags to place them in overnight.

Why clear? It's not likely that your bag will be mistaken for trash, given that it will be close to your tent and will be on the heavy side, but it's not worth chancing. None of the crew is likely to pick it up and toss it, but passersby may think, "Hey, trash bag!" and throw garbage in with it.

Since there is a significant chance that your bag will be outside all night, I also recommend using a small cable combination lock on the zipper. Just in case.

And an aside: the tents are cramped, but that's not a bad thing. With two people inside, their body heat helps warm it up, and with a bigger tent that's less heat surrounding you. My first year I had a tent to myself and I felt like I was freezing; the next year I had a tent mate, and it was much warmer even though the outside temperatures were lower.

But…it's your first night in camp, the tent is up, your mattress inflated (please don't wait until you're heading for bed to do this; some walkers go to sleep early and an air pump going off at even 8:30 is dismissive of their need for a little extra shut-eye) and you're ready to hit the showers.

Nope.

Now you need to go explore a little bit—go see the 3 Day Store, go see if you've gotten any mail, visit the remembrance tents, and eat. Don't even think about getting into the shower until after you've had some food and something to drink. In fact, if you've purchased towel service (and you want to do that) before they hand over your towels you'll be asked if you've eaten yet.

Don't lie; if you haven't, admit it. And then don't be offended when they won't give you your towels, but tell you to go eat first. They're not trying to be mean; too many people have passed out in the showers on day one because they were dehydrated and in need of food. And when you pass out in the showers, they will drag you out, bare-assed naked. They're not kidding when they say that. They *will* drag you out naked, wet, and completely unconscious.

So, eat before showering.

Unless you're into that kind of thing.

~

The food on the 3 Day in the last couple of years has been pretty good. When I walked in 2010, the Friday night non-vegetarian dinner was steak; it was damned tasty steak, too, and I wish I could have enjoyed it more, but that first walk day was a lesson in proper hydration for me. By the time I went through the food line and sat down to eat, I was nauseated and had to force myself to even cut into the steak. I managed to eat a little more than half, but I did drink quite a bit…and fifteen minutes later I was hungry.

Lesson learned.

Dinner on Saturday was grilled chicken with marinara sauce. Having food allergies and not knowing what was in the sauce, I opted to not have any, but the chicken was excellent without it. In fact, I didn't think I'd ever had chicken so good. Along with the veggies and bread and dessert, I killed dinner Saturday night.

I should point out that I made an effort to drink more on the second day, and am pretty sure that's why I had an appetite.

Breakfast is a buffet of scrambled eggs and the like; Saturday morning there were also muffins and Sunday there were danishes. I am not a morning person by any stretch of the imagination and in spite of everything I had promised myself pre-walk I just couldn't face breakfast, but the muffins and danishes were pre-wrapped and I took a couple to go.

In 2011, lessons learned about hydration, I ended each walk day with a hell of an appetite. Friday night was pasta with meatballs on the side, Greek salad, bread, and three different kinds of cake to choose from as dessert. Saturday was a citrus grilled chicken and potatoes – it was all either seriously good, or I am such a bad cook that it seemed incredible, so I had no complaints about the food.

In Atlanta I decided to force myself into eating breakfast. Thanks to my traveling companion, Michelle, I'd learned that I could eat scrambled eggs for breakfast and keep them down, so I opted for the eggs and a muffin in the morning. For assembly line eggs, they were pretty freaking tasty. I guarantee I don't make them as well at home.

Okay, so I am a bad cook.

Still.

The dining tent is where you might want to hang out in

the evening. After almost everyone has had a chance to grab dinner and eat, there's the camp show, karaoke, dancing (yes, after walking twenty miles, you might want to dance) and a game or two. It can be a hell of a lot of fun, so if you have the energy you might want to stick around for it.

Or, you might want to get that shower you've been longing for.

Showering is another common concern for first time walkers. *What are the shower trucks like? It is just one big open area where you watch each other get naked and then shower? Will I just want to skip it and stink?*

No worries. You will have the best two showers of your life in those trucks. And while previous versions of the shower trucks had a common area for changing, they had curtains around each shower stall. The current trucks have twelve showers stalls each and each stall has its own private changing area. So you'll be able to undress without an audience, shower as immodestly as you choose, and get dressed alone.

If you get there early enough you might not have to wait for a shower, but waiting an hour for the women's showers is not unheard of. There are fewer men on the walks and they usually only get one truck, or even just one half of a truck (six stalls are on each end) but the men don't typically have to wait as long as do the women.

Even if you wind up waiting, that hot shower will feel wonderful, and you'll be ready to hit the sack and face the next day.

DAY 2

The second day begins just as early as the first—the route tends to open (meaning they'll let you leave camp) around 7:30, but unlike the first day, you won't have to get up at four in the morning unless you want to or you have to pee (I'm guessing if you're up that early it's due to the latter; if you drank enough the day before, chances are you'll be getting up a couple of times at night to shuffle to the port-a-potties.) You'll have until 8:30 to get out onto the route; breakfast starts at 4 a.m. (most crew members get up *a lot* earlier than the walkers) so you have plenty of time to wake up, swear about being sore, take care of your feet, prep for blisters, get dressed, go eat, and breathe a little before starting out.

On day two you'll walk between nineteen and twenty one miles, and you might discover that unlike on day one when the thought that this all needs to be over soon hits you around mile sixteen, that it hits around mile eight. Day two can be the hardest of all three days; the first day you walk with a burst of excitement and energy, but day two can be when the negative thoughts creep in.

On the second day of my first walk, I was feeling pretty crappy by mile seven, and had the actual thought that this felt less like a charity walk and more like a death march. I was hot, I was miserable, my feet hurt, and I wanted to sit for a long, long time. By the time we got to lunch, I wasn't even sure how much longer I could go on.

As I got my sandwich, chips, and apple, the crew member handing them out asked how I was doing, and I was honest: *it's kind of sucking right now*. She smiled just a little and said she knew how that felt, but to bear in mind that the second day is almost always the hardest, and the closer I got to camp, the better I would feel.

Oh, and drink more.

I was drinking; I was drinking more than I did on the first day, but as we approached the next pit stop it occurred to me that I'd had more water than sports drink; I filled my bottle (crew guy manning the bottles: *what flavor ya want, orange, red, or purple?*) with purple, drank half, refilled it, and realized as we moved on that I did indeed feel better.

It *might* have been the Girl Scout cookies we'd been given at that pit stop.

Still, after hydration and cookies, things felt a lot better. I could feel just about every muscle in my body, and the balls of my feet felt like Moleskin-covered mush, but I'd gotten some energy back and felt pretty freaking good.

With about five miles to go, however, a hot spot on one foot was screaming and my (arthritically challenged) lower back was on fire, and with the next 3.5 miles being mostly up steep hills, my teammate Roberta strongly suggested I take the sweep van that was waiting right there.

It was a dilemma; I'd wanted to walk every step of the 3 Day, but a couple of things made me agree. One, I was slowing down and holding her back, and two, I wanted to be able to walk day three, and with my back as bad as it is, if I'd gone up hill all that way, day three was in doubt.

So I listened to my teammate and took the sweep van to the next pit stop.

No harm, no foul.

Day 3

Sunday morning is a little noisy in camp; it's a bit more than the chatter of Saturday morning, with tents unzipping as people crawl out to head for food or to pee. Sunday morning you have to pack up as you mutter about how all that stuff fit in the bag before, why won't it fit now? You need to deflate your mattress, shove it in your bag, eyeball the tarp and decide it doesn't need to go home, get everything else jammed in there and set outside the tent, which you must now take down and fit back into that tiny pink bag it came in.

If you look around, you'll probably see a few people so frustrated with the taking down of their tent that they just roll it up and try to jam it into the little bag (and not successfully) but it actually does fit if you do it right. Three simple steps:

1. After taking out the tent poles, fold the tent into quarters.
2. Roll the tent towards the tent door; this allows air to escape.
3. Collapse the tent poles and roll the tent around them.

It'll be nice and tight, and will slip into the bag and you'll be amazed at your camping skills.

Drag your bag and tent to the same place you picked them up from, stack the tent on the pile of other tents, hand your bag off to a crew member, and go eat.

Drink, too.

Drink, pee, no I.V.

~

Unless you're young and/or a freak of nature, on day three you're going to have sore feet, possibly sore calves, a sore back, and a sore neck. And chances are, you won't care. This is it, the last day of the walk. It will also be the shortest day, with the route being roughly sixteen miles long.

Why so short? Why not twenty?

Well…the first two days you likely walked more than twenty miles, and whether you realize it or not you have somewhere between forty-two and forty-four miles behind you. Plus, they need to get everyone done early enough to have closing ceremonies, and then time for everyone to get their gear and leave.

All in all you might walk only fifty-five miles. Or you might walk sixty-one. The route is as close to sixty as is possible in any given city, dependent on which streets and paths the 3 Day can get access to.

It really doesn't matter; you walked, you get to claim sixty.

The last day of the walk is the day when you just might cave into The Stupid. You know you "only" have sixteen miles or thereabouts, and you're determined to do them all, and to get done long enough before the closing ceremony so that you can sit around and talk to people, enjoy the atmosphere, take pictures, and have some fun.

That eagerness to finish fast can cost you.

You're going to be tired, you're going to be achy. You're also going to be pumped full of adrenaline because *this is it!* You might not think to drink enough, or you might skip the sports drinks because you're "only" doing sixteen miles and you don't want all that sodium and stuff bloating you later. It should be fine to skip the sports drink and avoid the salty snacks. Right?

Mistake. Big mistake.

Everything you've done to protect your body in training and on the first two days, you have to do on day three, and you may need to amp it up a bit. Be zealous in your foot care. Eat at least a little something at every pit stop. And more than anything, *drink*. And don't just drink water. Suck down the sports drink; at least half of all the liquids you consume, make it the sports drink.

I know this from experience.

On my third walk, in Atlanta, I was tired, achy, and determined to finish in spite of the fact that several of my medical issues were poking at me. I was drinking water, but I wasn't drinking nearly enough of the sports drink. A couple of miles before the lunch stop I was somewhat brain fogged, knew I need more to drink, and told myself that I would stop at lunch, check my feet and take care of the blister on my left foot, eat, drink, grab more to drink, and be on my way.

I got to lunch, sat down, checked my feet, added more Moleskin to pad the tender areas, drank some water…and then left.

I didn't get lunch.

I didn't get more sports drink to add to my water bottle.

I just got up and walked off.

If I had been doing what I was supposed to do all along, I would have had enough electrolytes on board to think clearly, and I would have had a clue as to why I was at the lunch stop. Food! Drink!

The fact that I didn't need to pee should have been a clue.

Two miles later, I caught up with a teammate who asked how I was doing, and I admitted, I was a little whipped. The guy on safety crew at the intersection we were waiting to cross also asked me how I was—that should have been a clue that I wasn't looking so hot to other people—and it was agreed that I should sit down for a few minutes, and if I was still feeling like that, he would get call for a sweep van.

Ten minutes and a little water later I thought I felt fine, and after all, there was a Grab-n-Go in about a mile.

I walk roughly a twenty-minute mile; it took me half an hour to reach the Grab-n-Go, which I simply passed. I noted it was there, but by then it didn't occur to me that I should stop. I kept right on walking, because there was a pit stop in a little less than three miles.

Between that Grab-n-Go and the next pit stop, I was asked by at least five people per mile if I was all right. Many of them were aware of my issues and the questions were practically patter:

How do you feel? Are you drinking? Have you had electrolytes? When was the last time you ate? What did you eat? Have you had any sugar? Any salt? Are you sure you're all right, because I can get you a sweep van.

I insisted I was fine.

That was stupid.

It was obviously not the truth; one fellow walker wouldn't go on ahead of me until I'd drained half of what was in my water bottle and accepted a couple of healthy slugs from his (I swear I have not backwashed!) sports drink. More than one person must have mentioned me to the crew at the pit stop, because when I got there a doctor who wouldn't let me brush off anything by mumbling, "I'm fine" greeted me at the pit stop entry. He grabbed me by the arm and steered me towards food, and wasn't happy until I'd gotten chips, fruit, and sports drink. I was ordered to sit in a folding metal chair near the medical tent and to rest, eat, and rehydrate.

I'm really not a stupid person; that was my third walk, I knew what I was supposed to do, but people, when you're that tired and you make a mistake early on, it can snowball on you.

Start doing it right from the very beginning of day three, so that you can make it to the holding area without getting red carded, or worse, put into the back of an ambulance to be taken to the emergency room.

Because holding? It's a blast.

~

Holding? They're going to hold me? How? Why? And what are they going to hold on me? After all that, I'm going to be *held?*

Yep.

But, it won't be against your will. You're free to come and go, but I guarantee you'll want to stay.

Somewhere around the last two miles, as excited as you'll probably be to see the end of the walk, you'll probably also have the stray thought—it might zip in and out, or it might take root—that you're never doing this again. It was awesome and you loved it, but once was enough. Next year, you're just going to raise money for someone else to walk.

That thought occurred to me toward the end of my first walk, and I heard it voiced from other people around me. *Hey, this was a great idea,* BUT.

This was a bucket list thing and I did it, and my friend who couldn't do it this year wants to do it next year, BUT.

My body held up and this didn't hurt nearly as much as I thought it would, BUT.

But…you haven't reached the end yet, and the moment you step into the holding area, you just might be dropping those Buts all over the place.

The first walkers who get into holding might not have the same WHOA feelings that the later walkers get, but they do get That Feeling (I've been a middle-of-the-pack arrival to holding and an early one, but not among the very first, so I'm guessing here.) Holding is essentially the last pit stop of the walk, and when you walk into holding, you're greeted by two lines of people wildly cheering you home. The early walkers are cheered in by crew members; the later walkers are cheered in by crew and their fellow walkers. Those two lines—you'll walk between them as you come in—will get several people deep. It's loud. It's energetic. And you may find yourself crying like a baby. Or cheering loudly right along with them. Or grinning so hard it feels like your face will crack. You may experience all of those and then some.

It is *the* definition of awesome.

You might even be tempted to go back outside and do it again.

Once you make it through the welcoming cheerleaders, head for the tent that says VICTORY SHIRTS and get your credentials scanned one last time, and collect your prize.

You did do it just to get the shirt, right?

I totally do it for the shirt.

After you have your shirt—and put it on!—take a moment to look around. Get your teammates together and take pictures at the sixty-mile sign. Go watch the people who still have so much energy they can't help but dance; seriously, after three days and sixty miles, people dance. Drink. Pee. Go cheer the walkers coming in after you.

Take a good look; you're going to want to take it all in, because that feeling you have, that's what's going to grab you. That's what will make you determined to do this again. And again. And again.

~

After the last walker has come home—don't laugh, in that moment it is truly a homecoming—the crew members are acknowledged and get the accolades they completely deserve while they walk through the lines of cheering walkers, and then everyone will be directed to line up, usually five to ten across, holding hands and locking arms as the entire group walks to the closing ceremony site.

Don't worry, it won't be far. I point that out because on my first walk, as we were all heading out, in spite of the excitement and wonder, I did allow the thought to zip through my head: we just walked sixty miles, how many more do they want?

It was just a couple of blocks. On my third walk I didn't

even think about it, but that one turned out to be an even shorter distance. Holding was at Turner Field in Atlanta, and we simply went to the parking lot.

No one is going to torture you with a surprise mile.

Closing is a lot like opening; the same stage, the same raised center island, and you cram in and get as close to the stage as you can. And before it really gets rolling you might even have a "let's just get this over so we can go home" thought.

Heck, I did.

On all three walks so far, that notion has zipped through my head.

But then it starts…really listen to the things being said. You'll be blown away at how much money your city raised, and you can't help but get excited about that.

And then, to put it bluntly, this chit gets real.

In front of and around you is a sea of white. Almost all of the walkers, proudly wearing the white victory shirts they earned. But then enters the mass of pink, the survivors. The women and men who have faced the disease we've walked against, women and men who have fought back and who have won.

Swallow now, because you might not able to for a while after that.

As the survivors come in, the shoes come off. Every walker takes off a single shoe and holds it high over his or her head. Your feet hurt, might even be swollen, but you'll take that shoe off in tribute to these people who have become warriors, and in memory of those who didn't make it.

The survivors join hands and raise their arms together as The Banner goes up, the flag that announces what we're all there for, what we all trained for, sweat for, bled for, cried for, and then walked for.

A world without breast cancer.

AFTER THE WALK HAS BEEN THOROUGHLY ROCKED

The walk is over; you're crawling into a real bed, still pumped up but looking forward to a long, quiet, full night's sleep, wrapped in the warmth of more than a sleeping bag and sweat pants.

You're done, right? No more pounding the pavement, no more stretching, no drinking copious amounts of water, no more sports drink.

Nope.

Chances are you're going to be a little sore after the walk; you'll need to keep stretching for a couple of days at least. And like it or not, you need to keep drinking, and ideally you're going to drink some of that sports drink as well.

Here's the thing...you've just put your body through a fairly traumatic three days. While you've been drinking enough to keep your electrolytes in balance and have been peeing a lot more than you ever thought you could, your muscles are holding onto quite a bit of that water. Muscles under stress tend to do that; you're drinking and peeing, using the amount of urine and its color as an indicator to how well hydrated you are, but your muscles are holding onto a good part of what you consumed all weekend.

This is also why you might not want to get on a scale for a few days; you're probably going to have gained a few pounds over the weekend, and it's not just because you ate your way from opening to closing ceremonies. It's because those traumatized muscles are holding water, and they're not going to let go of it until they're convinced everything is all right. It could be anywhere from three pounds to ten pounds, and you need to convince those muscles to shed the fluid.

How?

Drink. Not just water, but replace the electrolytes you'll be flushing out as well. It sounds counterintuitive, but by staying on top of the hydration, your body will let the extra water weight go.

Yep. *Drink, pee, no IV* still applies.

(And the post-walk Long Island Iced Tea and tequila shots don't count.)

~

There are a lot of tongue-in-cheek post-walk jokes; you go for a walk and hear a car horn and immediately turn and wave, embarrassed because it wasn't for you. You're out and about and stop to tie your shoe and are surprised because no one else stopped to make sure you're all right. You're in the middle of a crowd waiting to cross a busy street at an intersection and can't understand why you're the only one stretching.

I find the post-walk hyperbole amusing; and that's really all it is, tongue-in-cheek ways of expressing some of the awesome that happens on the walk that you just don't tend to get in everyday life. I've never thought a honking car was for me; I've never stretched at a busy intersection because I was still in walking groove.

It would be really funny, though, even if to no one else but me.

Still, after participating in a 3 Day you'll probably realize, as you're walking along a busy downtown street, passing by hundreds of other people, that a great number of them will soon be diagnosed with breast cancer. You might start counting the women you pass, and be stabbed with the thought that every eighth one will face that diagnosis this year alone. It might be overwhelming, and you might need to stop and suck in a deep breath.

As you wander through your real life and those numbers start feeling very real, remember, too, that in the multitude of people you pass, many of them have walked the walk, too. They know what the effort you went through feels like, they know what it takes, and like you, they're changed. And they will likely do another walk in the future.

But all those other people, the strangers you'll never know, the people who are going about their daily business and not thinking about what the next day, the next hour, or the next minute might bring, most of them are people who absolutely would honk for you. They would make sure you're all right if they thought there was any question. They would stretch right along with you, if they thought it would make you feel any less weird about it.

People do care about the effort you made. You didn't do it for the accolades; you didn't have focusing attention on yourself on your mind, other than the amount of it you needed to grab for fundraising, and your expectations were not more than contributions from friends and family. The further from the walk you get, the less of a big deal it might seem.

You did it; you'll probably do it again.

No big deal, right?

Keep looking at the people you pass by; really look at them. If they knew, they would understand what a big deal it is. Most of them can't even comprehend trying to walk twenty miles in one day, much less sixty in three. Most of them would understand something very fundamental: you don't know them, but what you did—all the training, the sweat, the tears, the blisters and the blood—you did it for something that might happen to them, and it matters.

One out of every eight women, every year.

1,500 men diagnosed, and between 400 and 500 will die every year.

Every year.

But.

BUT.

You walked; you raised money. Every dime you squeezed out of other people will make a difference, and to a random stranger, it might mean life.

None of those people know what you accomplished, but if they did, they would have one thing to say, one thing you probably heard a lot on the walk but not much afterward. One thing you deserve to hear, because your efforts *will* save someone else's life. But they don't know, and they can't say it to you, so I will.

Thank you.

From the bottom of my heart, thank you.

TIPS

Fundraising Tips

Be willing to do just about anything; I agreed to ride a motorcycle through a very popular outlet mall, dressed in pink spandex and a pink cape in exchange for the donation of an iPad to be used as a donor prize. Later, I spent a day walking around San Francisco in the same getup, along with a pink fedora; I had to wander not just in the areas where pink spandex doesn't draw a second look, but where the tourists migrate toward as well, and that netted me $1000 in donations. For my second walk that year, I dyed my hair neon pink and walked in pink camo pants for $400.

Hold a yard sale; get rid of your unwanted junk and use the proceeds to self-fund part of your goal. Bonus: not only are you getting rid of things taking up valuable house space, but what you self-donate is tax deductible.

Don't limit yourself when asking people to donate. If you say, "even ten dollars will help" you'll probably only get ten dollars. If you're uncomfortable hitting up friends for $100, then phrase it differently; point out that if X number of people each donate $100, it only takes Y amount of donations to reach your goal. And remind everyone that their donations are tax deductible.

The phrase "tax deductible" makes a difference to some potential donors, and they may donate more if they understand it's a tax-time writeoff.

Some local restaurants will host fundraising events for you; as long as you get the word out and make coupons available, they'll give you an evening where they donate X% of the tab on coupon holders' purchases. Frozen yogurt stores often host a block of time where all anyone has to do is say that they're there for the fundraiser, and you get 10-15%.

Grocery stores will often allow people to set tables up outside their doors; create some colorful posters, get a giant tip jar for people to shove change and dollar bills into, and set up. It helps to have flyers available stating what you're doing, why, with all the pertinent statistics. You can hand out stickers and candy, too.

Check out other potential hot spots, like the gym, big box retailer, library, etc. Ask permission first, but many will allow you to have a table outside the front door.

Bake sale (local laws permitting).

Car wash: get your kids and friends involved, and host a donations-requested car wash. Many stores with available outside water will allow fundraising car washes in their parking lots.

Use social media: don't be afraid to post weekly to Facebook, Twitter, your blog, or any other media. Ask for donations, leave a convenient link to your fundraising page. I get most of my donations via my cat's blog. Seriously.

Packing tips

Pack *everything* in ziplock baggies; that way if your bag happens to get wet, your clothing and other things will stay dry. Use 2 gallon ziplock bags for clothing; once the clothes are in the bag, zip it closed except for about an inch, and then squeeze all the air out. Then finish zipping it up. That helps compact your clothing.

Use a sharpie marker to write Friday, Saturday, Sunday on the bags; that makes it easier to keep track and NOT wind up grabbing the previous day's dirty underwear.

Don't pack more than you'll need. Your bag needs to be 35 pounds or less, and that includes your sleeping bag and air mattress. You can walk in the same t-shirt and shorts or pants for 3 days; it might stink a little by the end of the third day, but everyone else is going to smell, too, so that really doesn't matter.

To get a good idea if you're taking too much stuff, everything other than your mattress, sleeping bag, the shoes you'll wear on day one, backpack or waist pack, and jacket should fit into a paper grocery bag.

If you're bringing a battery operated air pump, don't put the batteries in it in the right direction; put them in backwards. That way if the switch gets nudged on the pump while it's in your bag, it won't drain. For the same reason, don't use a rechargeable pump; I learned that the hard way on my first walk.

For tarps, get the thin plastic painting dropcloths. Those are cheap and they're very light.

Bring something you can place outside your tent at night to help you find your tent in the dark. Pink is not a great idea; the tents are pink and lots of people bring pink. Anything but pink. You can even use a cheap, colorful shower curtain on your tent; just make sure you use plenty of clothespins to pin it to the tent so that it doesn't flap around in the breeze, annoying nearby walkers.

Don't bring a hair dryer. There's no place to plug it in, and the noise would annoy sleeping walkers, anyway.

Tips for Camp

A flashlight is helpful, because chances are you'll be walking around after dark or will have to get up in the middle of the night to pee. I recommend a head lamp instead of a hand-held flashlight. The head lamps are much more convenient in the port-a-potties when it's dark. Plus, you're less likely to drop it into a toilet.

If you do drop something into a port-a-potty, consider it gone. You're never getting it back. So you might not want to use your smart phone as a flash light, just in case.

Flip flops make for very good shower shoes.

Pay for towel service; that way you don't have to have the added weight of a towel and don't have to worry about how to dry it out after its first use on Friday night. You *will* need to bring your own washcloth, however.

If you're sharing a tent with your spouse...those tents are very thin and sound carries. Just something to think about.

Earplugs. Camp can be noisy and your tentmate might snore.

Think about the people around you in regards to sound; it's not party central in camp, so leave the booze at home (yes, this has been an issue) and don't sit up late giggling and gossiping. If you want to drink and have loud fun, you might want to stay in a hotel instead.

Put the bag with the clothes you're going to wear the next day in your sleeping bag so that they're nice and warm in the morning.

Self heating body wraps make for wonderful personal heaters in your sleeping bag.

General Tips

If you didn't use it during training, don't use it on the walk; this is not the time to test out new things.

If you're walking in a city you're unfamiliar with, check the weather forecast and pay attention to the average temps. It might be hot during the day and very cold at night, and you want to be prepared for both.

While you're not allowed to wear ear plugs or earphones, you can still have music. Bring a battery operated speaker to hang from your waistpack or backpack. You can still have music, and the walkers around you will enjoy it, too.

Second Skin is your friend; if you get a blister, this little moist square, covered by Moleskin or a blister bandage, can make it bearable.

Bring a lancet to drain blisters, and alcohol wipes to disinfect it. If a blister gets too big and you're too far from a pit stop, you might want to be able to drain it. This is not necessarily a *great* idea, but sometimes blisters just get too big to walk on, and draining them can be a relief.

Start using an anti-chafing power or stick early on in your training. Body Glide, Vaseline, and specific foot and body powers can keep the chafing at bay.

Make sure your sports bra fits snugly to prevent bleeding nipples. Guys, use something like Body Glide on yours. Your shirt rubbing on them all day can cause major chafing and bleeding, and once that happens, it hurts.

Moisture wicking underwear. Seriously.

Get your shoes a half size bigger than your normal street shoes. Your feet will swell on long walks, and you want to accommodate for that. Otherwise, you may lose a toenail or two after the walk. Or you may be cutting the toe box of the shoe off during the walk to make room for the swelling.

NO COTTON SOCKS! You want moisture wicking socks; there are dozens of brands available, so try out a couple early on to find out which ones you prefer.

Give Biofreeze a try on aching muscles and feet. It's just menthol, but it works quite well on taking the edge off muscle pain. Ben Gay and Icy Hot work well, too, but I recommend against Capsaicin cream unless you're going to use it AFTER you shower and are dry. It feels extra-hot when wet.

Make sure your lip balm has an SPF protectant. You don't want sunburned lips.

Sunglasses. Sunscreen. Seriously.

If it's cold in the morning, those extra socks you have make for nice mittens.

If more than one person has asked you in a fifteen-minute period if you're all right, consider that you might not look all right. Do an honest assessment of your condition.

Embrace the sweep van if needed. There is no shame in taking one; it's not the end of your walk, just a couple miles to get you to the next pit stop where you can rest.

There probably won't be anywhere to plug your cell phone in to recharge, so bringing a portable battery charger might be a good idea. You can get one for about $30, and it will last all weekend if all you charge is your phone.

Wear a hat; sunburned scalps suck, and after a while it will be agonizing.

The crew works hard to make the walk possible; don't forget to thank them.

Walk your own walk; it doesn't matter if people are passing you.

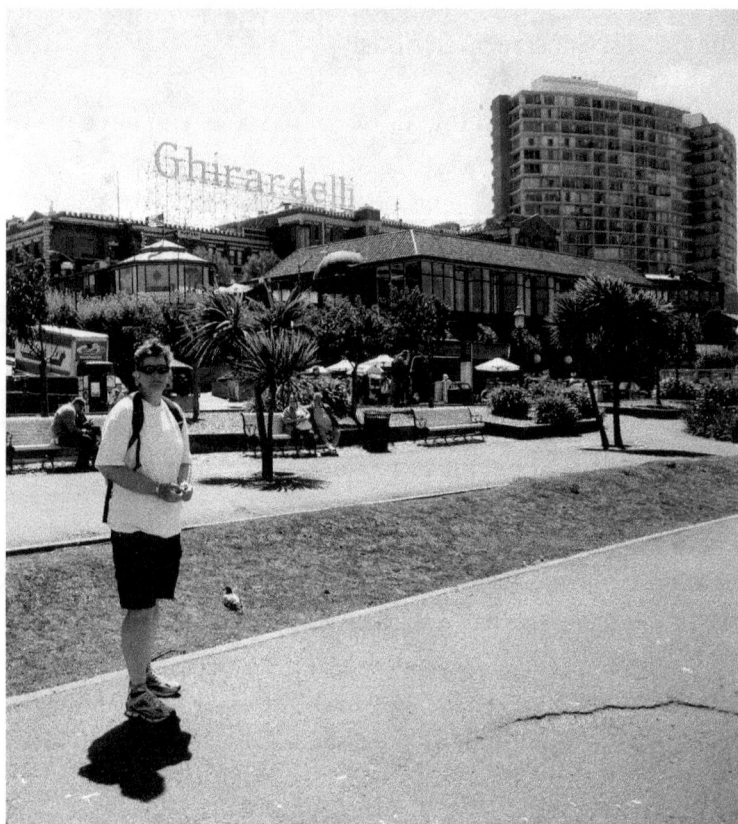

If you have fun places for your training walks, head for them...scenery beats walking around neighborhoods where the sights never change.

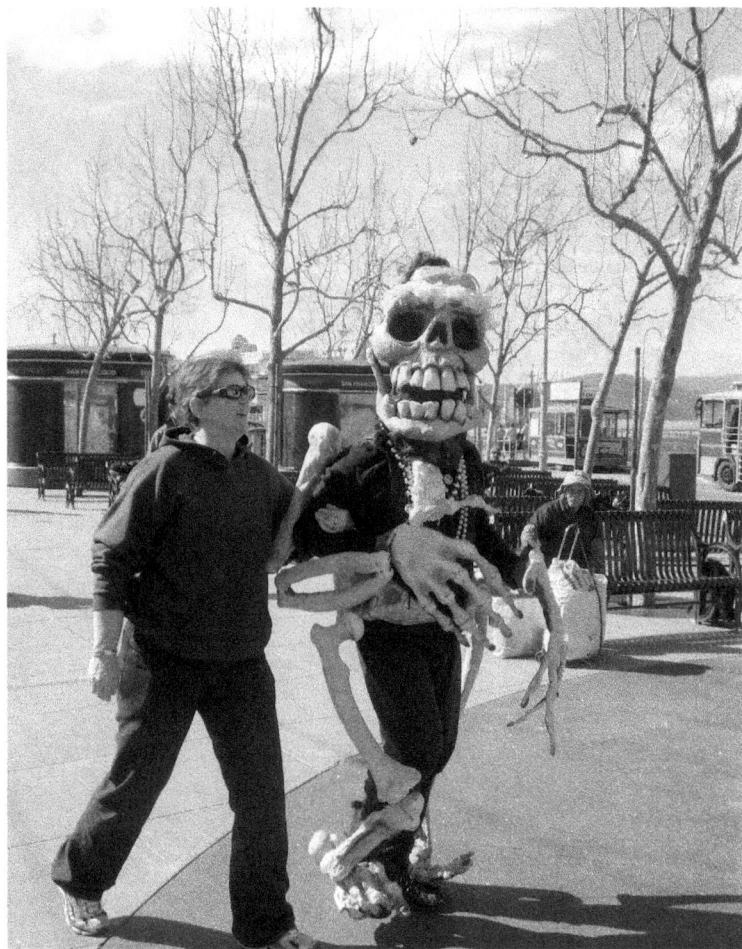

And hey, you never know who'll you'll meet along the way.

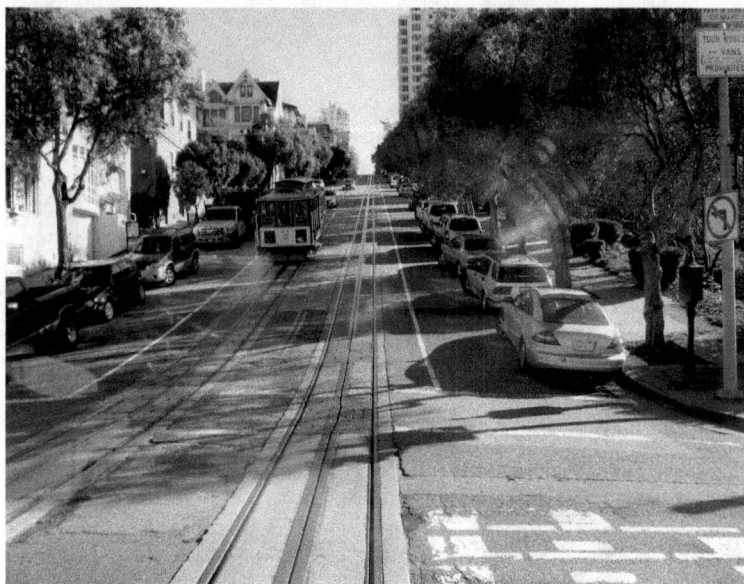

Hills. Train on them.

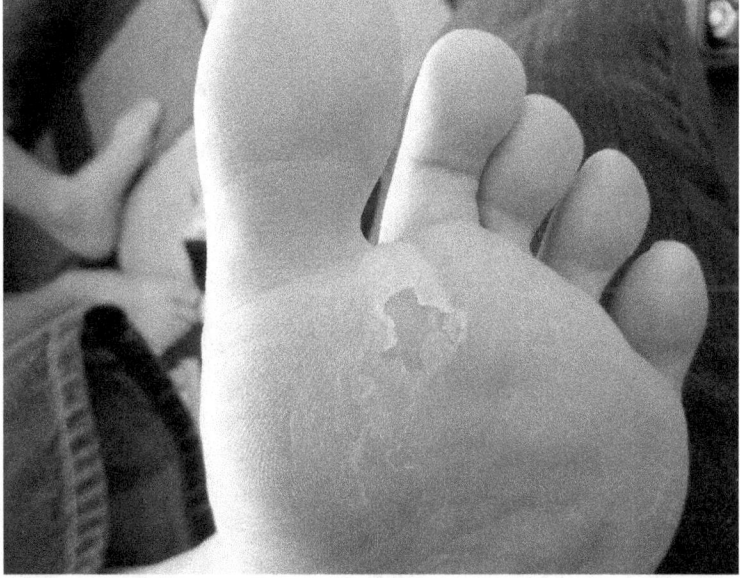

A blister under a blister...take care of your feet!

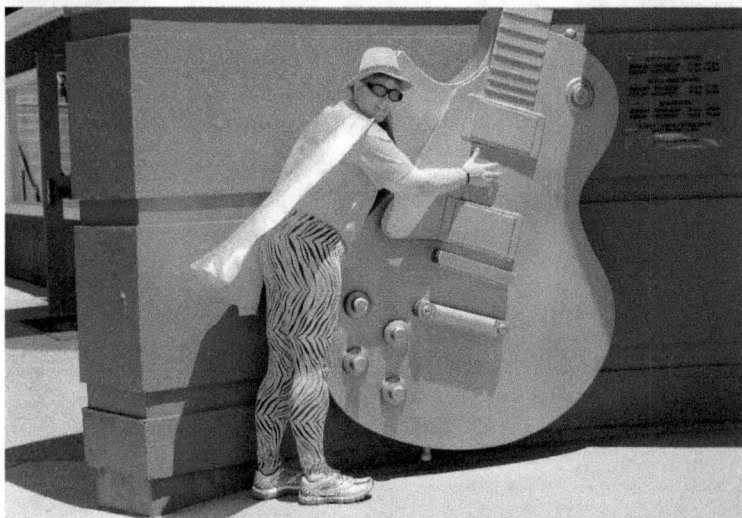

Yep, you'll do almost anything for donations. Pink spandex. In San Francisco, in front of the Hard Rock Cafe.

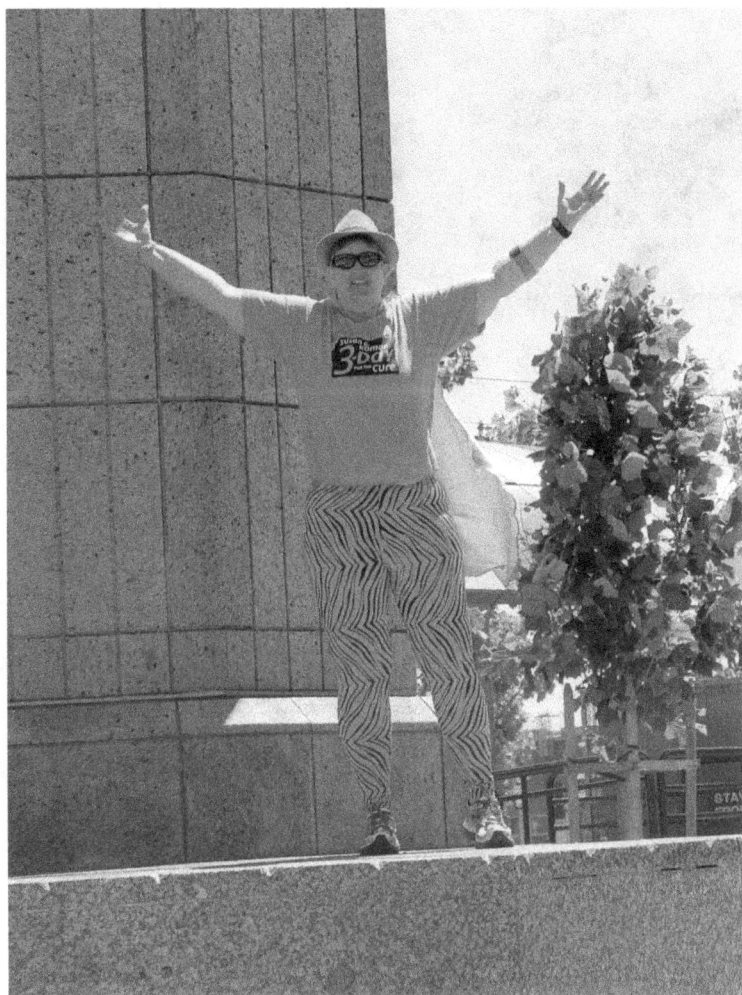

And on the Embarcaderro, at a majorly busiy intersection.

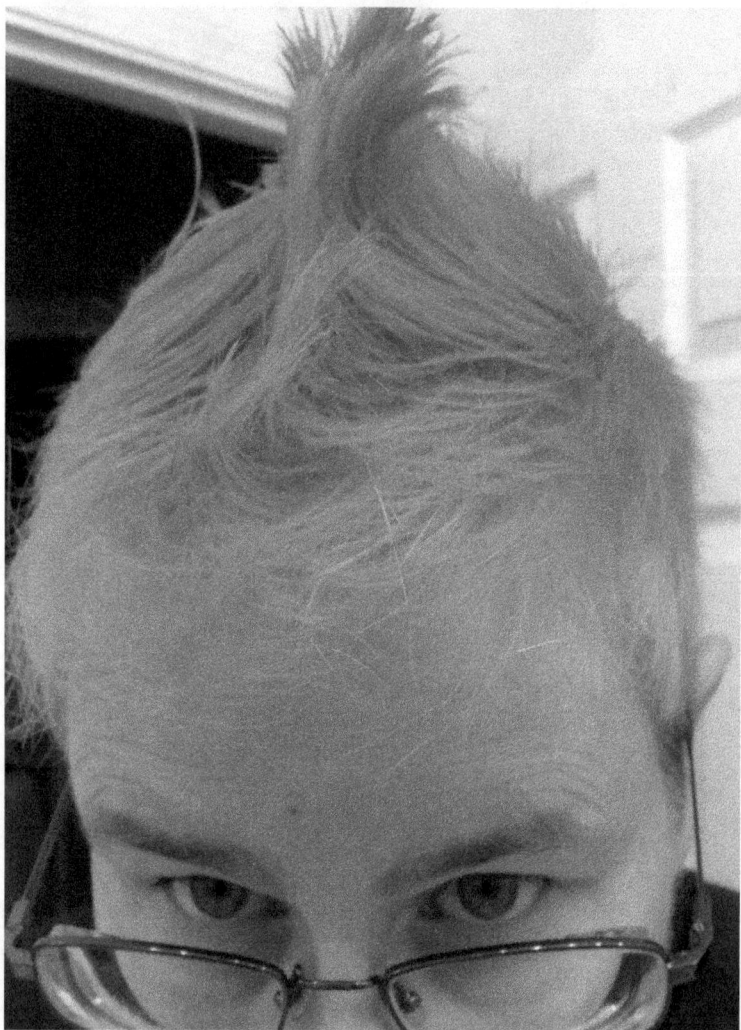

Hot pink fauxhawk...I'd be lying if I didn't admit that I kind of liked the pink hair...

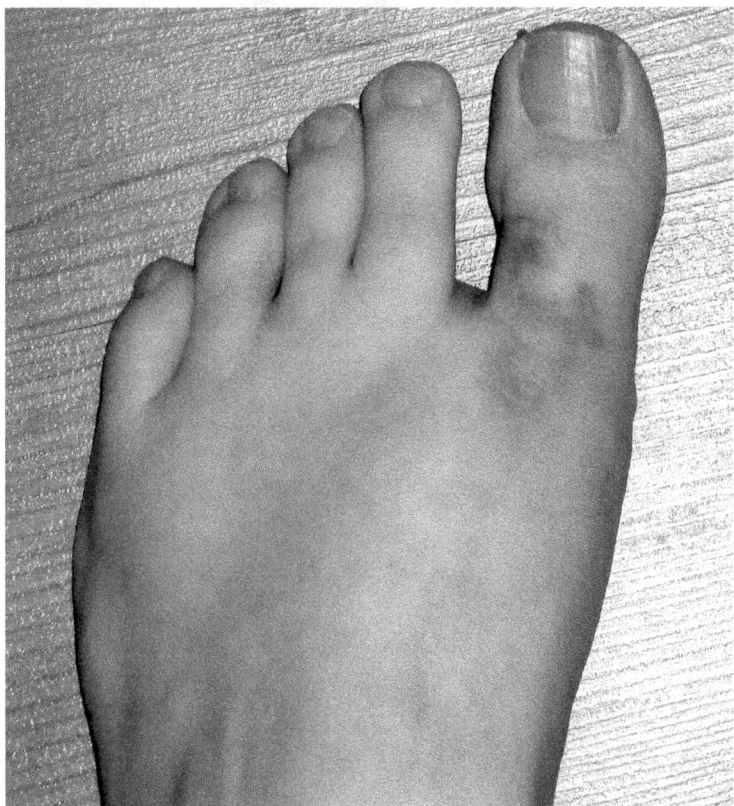

What you don't want to do: one week before the walk, break your big toe. That made for a fairly ouchy experience

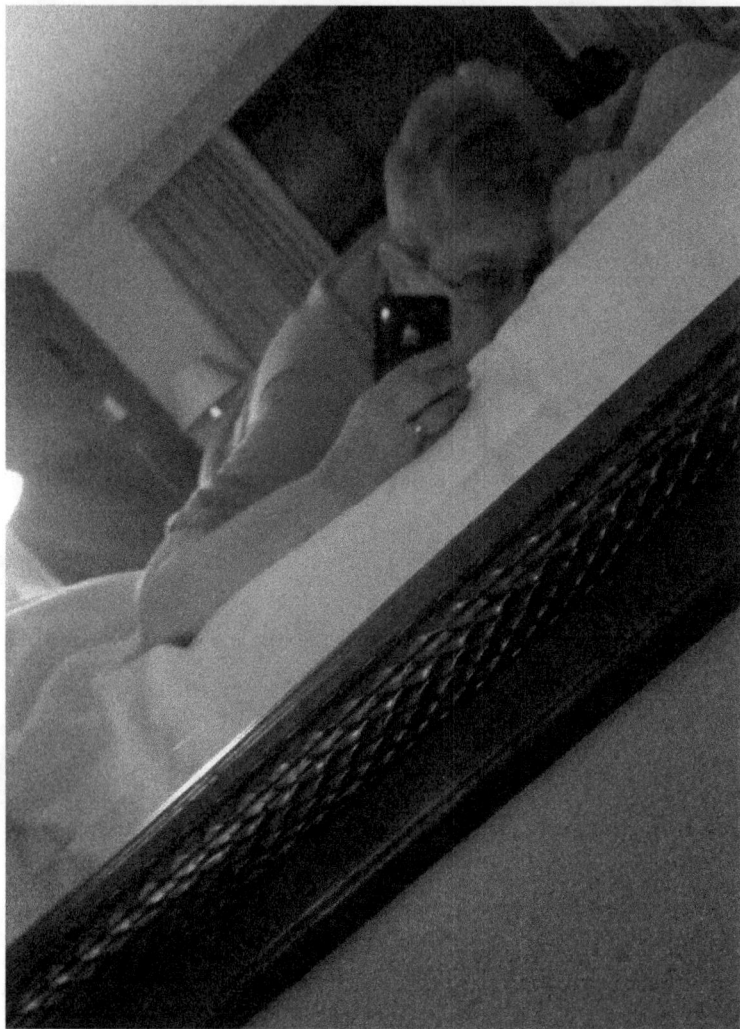

Four in the morning comes way, way too early...

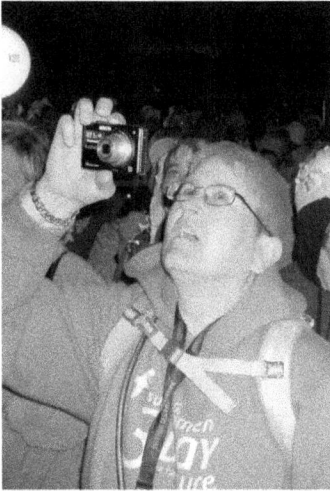

Take pictures!

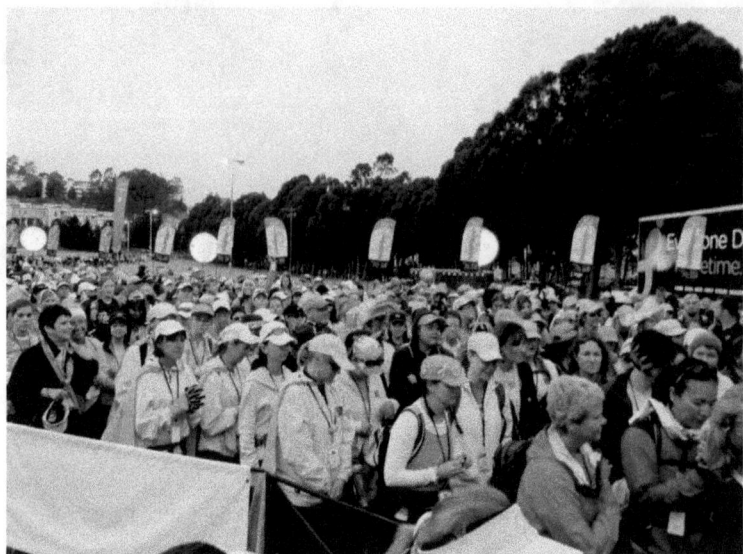

Opening ceremonies are a little crowded, but awesome.

And the memorial flag is amazing.

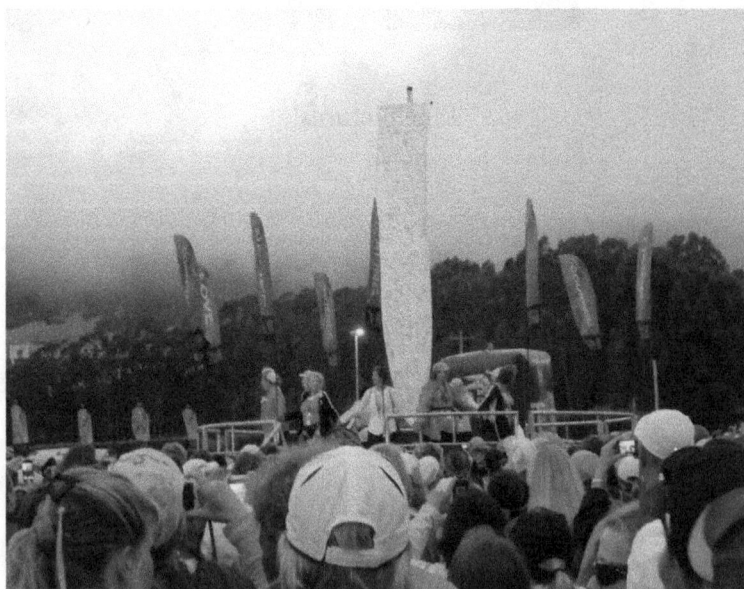

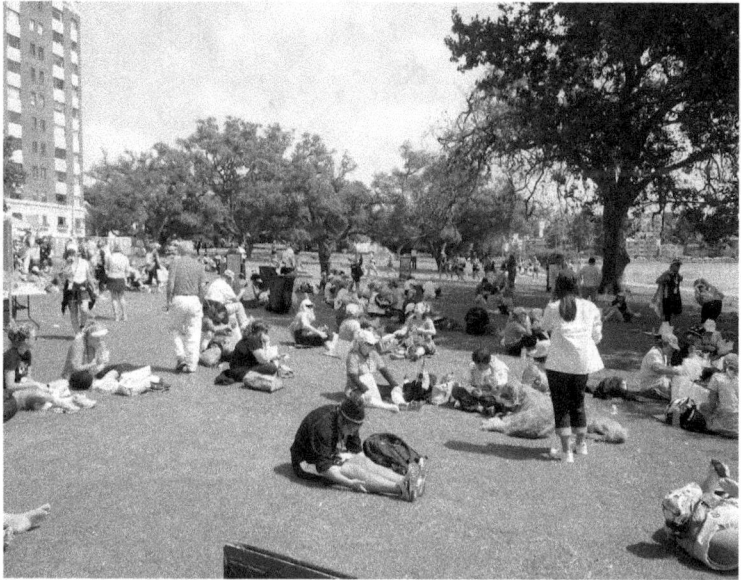

Lunch on the 3 Day.
Yep, chances are you'll be sitting on the ground.

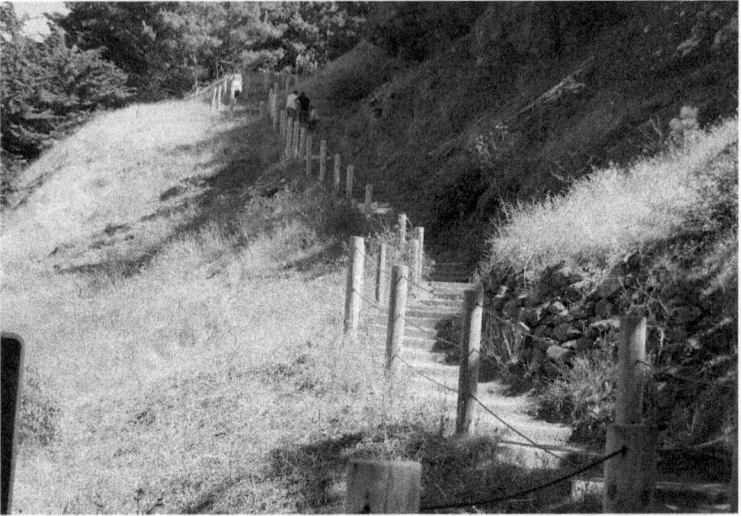

The Land's End stairs in San Francisco; 133 steps that tend to feel like 500. Don't worry, you can do it...just remember to train for stairs, like you train for hills. You may be ascending a few.

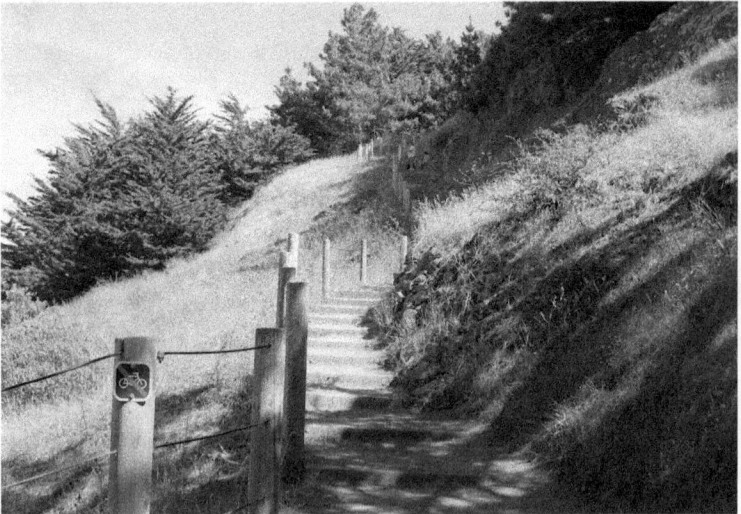

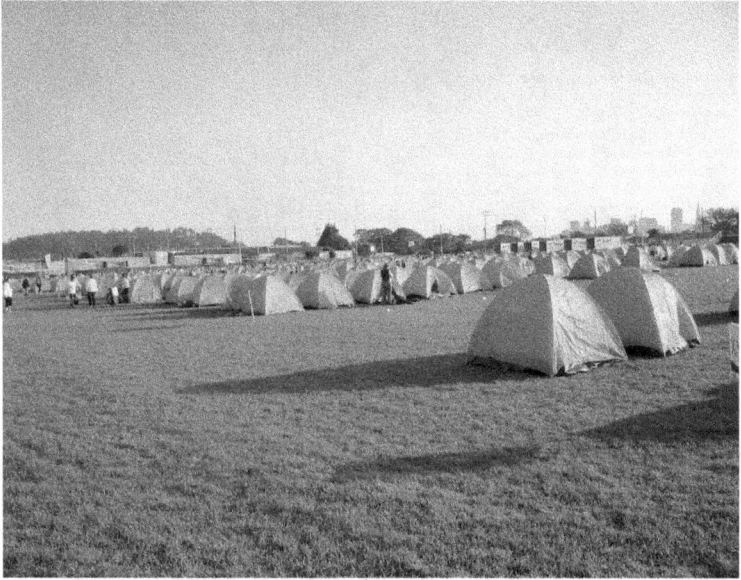

Camp is a sea of pink tents - this is early on, when fewer than half had been set up. It's a heck of a sight when everyone has their tent erected.

And the shower trucks...the most amazing shower ever.

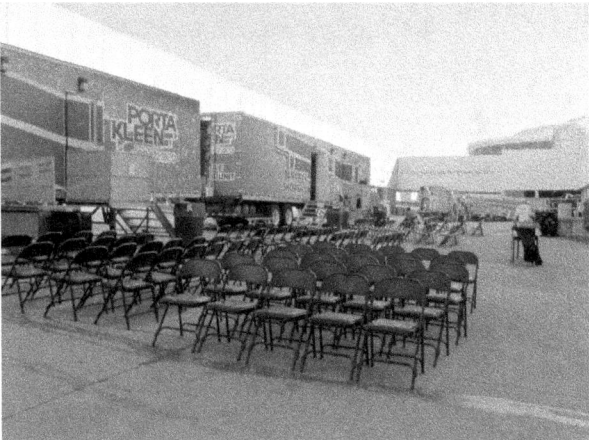

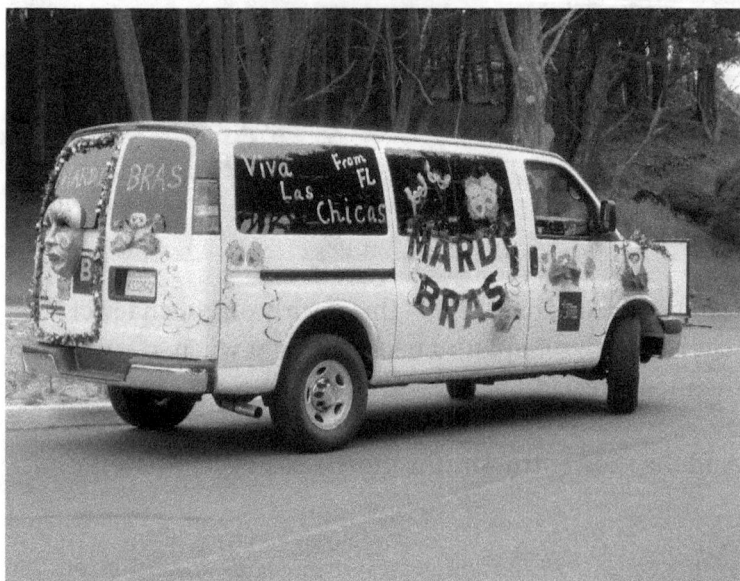

Embrace the sweep van if you need it! Fun things happen in the sweep van!

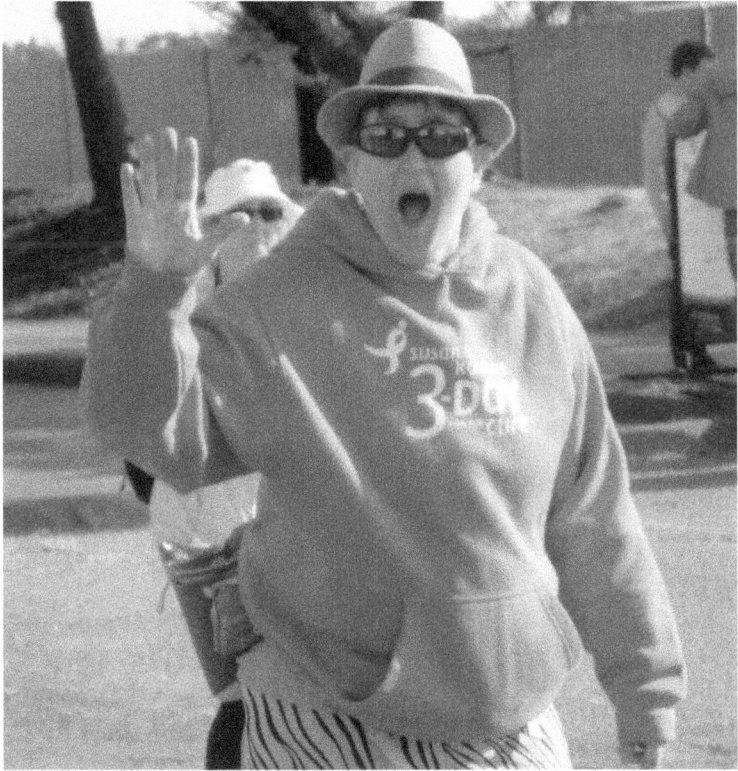

You're going to have a blast.
Rock the Walk while you Rock the Pink!

www.ingramcontent.com/pod-product-compliance
Lightning Source LLC
Chambersburg PA
CBHW050350280326
41933CB00010BA/1409